National Public Health and Hospital Institute
(NPHHI)

Managed Care and the Inner City

Dennis P. Andrulis
Betsy Carrier

Managed Care and the Inner City

The Uncertain Promise for Providers, Plans, and Communities

Jossey-Bass Publishers • San Francisco

Portions of Chapters 1, 2, and 3 were previously published in D. Andrulis, *The Urban Health Penalty: New Dimensions and Directions in Inner-City Health Care*. Public Policy Paper 1. Philadelphia: American College of Physicians, 1997. Reprinted with permission.

Jossey-Bass books and products are available through most bookstores. To contact Jossey-Bass directly, call (888) 378-2537, fax to (800) 605-2665, or visit our website at www.josseybass.com.

Substantial discounts on bulk quantities of Jossey-Bass books are available to corporations, professional associations, and other organizations. For details and discount information, contact the special sales department at Jossey-Bass.

 Lyons Falls Turin Book. This paper is acid-free and 100 percent totally chlorine-free.

Library of Congress Cataloging-in-Publication Data

Andrulis, Dennis P.
  Managed care and the inner city : the uncertain promise for providers, plans, and communities / Dennis P. Andrulis, Betsy Carrier.
      p. cm.
  Includes bibliographical references and index.
  ISBN 0-7879-4623-0 (hbk. : alk. paper)
  1. Managed care plans (Medical care)—United States.   2. Urban poor—Medical care—United States.   I. Carrier, Betsy.
II. National Public Health and Hospital Institute.   III. Title.
RA413.5U5A57   1999   98-56051
362.1'04258'0973—dc21   CIP

FIRST EDITION
HB Printing   10 9 8 7 6 5 4 3 2 1

Contents

Preface

Health care in the inner city is at a critical turning point. By 1998 the proportion of the employed population receiving health services under some sort of managed care had grown to 85 percent, up from 50 percent in only four years ("Health Insurers Seek . . . ," 1998). This sharp increase of managed care in commercial markets is spilling over into government-sponsored health insurance, with increasing numbers of individuals in the Federal Employees Health Benefit Program, Medicare, and Medicaid now being covered by managed care plans. At the same time, more and more urban hospitals, clinics, and community physicians who seemed immune from competition and the marketplace are falling under its sway. In fact, short-term acceleration into prominence has made managed care a primary force driving the delivery of health care to rich and poor alike across the United States. This growing influence of managed care on the way people get their health care and who provides that care means that the health of residents in America's urban areas will be increasingly affected by its presence.

Interestingly, these dynamics are occurring just as managed care itself is undergoing its own evolution. In the early 1990s managed care plans began cutting health care costs by 10 to 15 percent per year in the commercial market. This success led policymakers, payers, plans, and providers to ask whether managed care could have the same impact in other areas. Consequently they looked to government purchasers—Medicare and Medicaid—to manage care as a way to cut their costs. At the same time physician and hospital providers were experiencing a reduction in commercial revenues and seeking new sources of revenues. These circumstances caused health plans to enter the Medicaid and Medicare markets assertively. A recent headline reads, "The Fastest Growing Market in Healthcare Was . . . Medicare and Medicaid Risk Products" (Jacobs, 1996, p. 30). The excitement over these markets resulted in aggressive marketing that moved many Medicaid recipients and Medicare beneficiaries into managed care quickly. Enrollment in Medicaid managed care plans soared from 6.7 percent of total recipients in 1991 to 47.8 percent in 1997, or 15.3 million lives (Page, 1998). The number of Medicare beneficiaries in health maintenance organizations (HMOs) has more than doubled since 1995, reaching 5.2 million individuals, or over 12 percent of this population. In this book, most references to managed care refer to programs implemented under Medicaid.

In addition to this financial expansion, managed care itself is changing. For many years, its definition was almost synonymous with *health maintenance organization*. Although managed care plans tend to share several common features, including enrolling patients, contractual arrangements between provider and payer or purchaser of care, and medical management, the term *managed care* now encompasses a broad range of health delivery and financing arrangements intended to reduce cost and ensure the provision of care at the most appropriate site (Rowland, Rosenbaum, Simon, and Chait, 1995). These arrangements are likely to continue shifting, given the added weight of consumer concern and preferences for choice.

Both threat and opportunity lie ahead for inner-city residents in the evolving scenario of managed care and its various forms. The threat is that individuals who are working poor or low income, who historically have found quality health care difficult to obtain, could be alienated further from the health care system of middle-class America. The great opportunity is that managed care's success in the inner city could bring about a major break from the past fragmented, patchwork way of getting health care, replacing it with a substantially more far-reaching system of care for these communities. No clear direction has emerged to date.

Fundamental questions in current discussions command center stage. How can managed care and urban-based health service providers balance the financial objectives of achieving cost containment in health care with the societal goal of delivering quality health care and protecting vulnerable populations in the nation's inner cities? How can communities, governments, and the private sector play a role in creating what is best for their neighborhoods and cities?

Finally, health care system changes and market orientation discussions have also drawn attention to a group of inner-city providers that have traditionally been the mainstay for care to vulnerable populations. This group, often referred to as the health care safety net, consists of public and some private hospitals that provide a large amount of care to underserved and uninsured individuals, health centers or community clinics, and departments of public health. Together, they share two basic missions: to furnish comprehensive care to these populations and to provide a range of important screening, primary, and high-cost specialty services, such as trauma care, for which they frequently do not receive adequate compensation from insurers and patients. Great uncertainty also remains over what the dominance of managed care means for the future of the urban safety net.

The purpose of this book is to bring to light and discuss the dynamics around managed care and the inner-city providers that could create better health care for these populations—or could worsen an already difficult situation. It does this with the following objectives in mind. First, it considers for managed care professionals and more general audiences the environment and needs of inner-city communities, especially the working poor and other low-income residents; in so doing, it identifies how these needs are not currently being addressed and how they could be met. Second, it discusses and raises questions for concerned citizens, managed care organizations, and those in influential positions at the local, state, and national levels about the fit of managed care in the inner city— that is, how well it has addressed the needs of these communities to date; in weighing inner-city needs, it also identifies the value of traditional providers of inner-city care. Third, it describes the different organizational cultures surrounding these providers and managed care. It documents the adjustments being made by traditional providers of care within these cities generally, but focuses attention on the challenges of adaptation facing urban teaching hospitals, a sector that offers highly specialized care for rich and poor alike and is also a primary provider of care to inner-city residents. The conclusions drawn from the information suggest that successful transition through capitalizing on the strengths that both managed care and traditional providers bring to the inner city could lead to success for the health care system and communities; alternatively, failure could create even further service dysfunction. Finally, it discusses the financial influences in this evolution; the book offers to managed care organizations and agencies charged with the responsibility of financing and guiding the health system recommendations on how to create effective, sustainable services to the nation's inner cities.

The unsettled and changing nature of health care required that we consider both historical and current experiences, documenting problems as well as promising approaches. In addition, it was essential that we incorporate the views of managed care, inner-city communities, providers of health care, and government. To address the questions and objectives fairly and effectively while accounting for these perspectives, we chose to develop information from several sources. We conducted an extensive review of literature from journals, other formally published reports, testimony, and information releases from research and policy organizations. To provide a profile of inner-city health and health-related challenges, we obtained data from national sources, such as the Bureau of the Census, the FBI's Uniform Crime Reports, and the Centers for Disease Control and Prevention. We conducted structured interviews with directors of community-based managed care programs, health service research and policy professionals, and physicians. The purpose of these interviews was to obtain descriptions of health services and their organizations' functioning in inner-city settings, including the impact of new managed care and financing changes; to identify federal and state managed care–related actions and their effects on the inner city; and to document the experience of providers treating inner-city populations and coping with the changing environment. A fourth major source of information targeted urban teaching hospitals. We created, disseminated, and analyzed data from a 1997 national survey of these hospitals, requesting information on how managed care and the current marketplace were affecting their financial status, teaching activities, organization, staffing, and services. This survey also asked how these institutions were responding to managed care and implications of their adjustments.

The chapters in this book are organized to present the urban context and its challenges: how managed care has evolved to date in these settings, as well the relationship with providers who have been in these cities and health care financing concerns. Chapter One considers the complexity of the inner city—the characteristics of residents, including their racial and ethnic diversity, housing, poverty, and social factors. Integral to this review is the host of health conditions afflicting these individuals and the issues affecting their access to and use of health services. It emphasizes the importance of taking these characteristics into account in the organization and provision of health services.

Chapter Two discusses how managed care organizations and traditional providers of care to inner-city residents, especially low-income and vulnerable populations, currently address the needs of urban communities. Documented evidence to date highlights the potential benefits of managed care programs and promising initiatives designed for residents in these areas. However, the chapter cites recent studies that question whether managed care programs as currently configured can effectively address the health concerns of vulnerable populations. Additional review considers the historic role of the traditional providers of care in inner-city communities to both insured and uninsured. It suggests that their long-term experience is a potentially valuable, if not essential, asset for managed care organizations and may be vital for historically disenfranchised populations in these areas.

Chapter Three presents a review of the organizational cultures of managed care and the inner-city safety net providers. In so doing it points out similarities and differences in mission, system sophistication, financial incentives, staff composition, and status of their core support structures such as information systems. It suggests that the fit of these characteristics from the managed care and safety net perspectives is most often challenging, if not perilous, citing closures, financial hardships, and other consequences resulting from marketplace and managed care influences. Responses to these pressures are also addressed, with the objective of keeping core elements of the safety net while facilitating an effective managed care–provider relationship in urban settings.

Chapter Four uses the issues identified in the previous chapter to present how managed care is affecting urban teaching hospitals. Using results from the national survey, it portrays a provider group with great potential and benefit to its communities, but one that is struggling to change. The narrative discusses market shifts and managed care impact on revenues, efforts to recast services toward primary care, shifts among resident numbers, and other staff downsizing and adjustments.

Managed care's focus on cost containment and efficiency greatly influences the providers' direction, while the routes that inner-city health organizations and individuals take may determine whether they thrive or even survive. Chapter Five identifies how controlling revenues through incentives and disincentives may create particular problems for providers who are caring for inner-city populations. Using the experience of Medicaid managed care to date, it presents information suggesting that adjustments may not be sufficient to encourage delivery of high-quality, comprehensive services in these areas, with financial instability creating additional uncertainty.

Although initiatives identified in this chapter bring some promise of effective integration of a safety net role with the objectives of managed care, our conclusions reinforce the fragility of many safety net providers and the stark fact that little has been accomplished in incorporating the millions of uninsured into these organizational initiatives.

The final chapter draws on the collective experiences and information presented in previous chapters to suggest next steps and actions to create an effective, managed care–based system for inner-city communities. These recommendations are directed toward influential agencies and organizations such as federal and state governments, using the powers of financial incentive and regulation; private sector responsibilities to the populations in need; safety net providers to create the relationship with managed care organizations that is best for the communities in these urban settings; and managed care organizations to account for the broad social and health needs of inner-city residents. The conclusion calls for a national strategy to monitor the effect of managed care on the health and well-being of residents in inner cities across the United States.

February 1999   Dennis P. Andrulis
                                                                          New York

                                                                          Betsy Carrier
                                                                          Washington, D.C.

Acknowledgments

Financial support from the Center for Health Care Strategies made this book possible. We express our special appreciation to Yoku Shaw-Taylor and Rebecca Gold at the National Public Health and Hospital Institute for their extensive background work on this book. We thank the staff at the Association of American Medical Colleges, especially Robert Dickler, Ernest Moy, David Witter, and Kevin Serrin, for their assistance with the national survey on managed care and teaching hospitals. We are grateful to the individuals we interviewed including: Eric Baumgartner, Texas Department of Health; Maura Bluestone, Bronx Health Plan; Steve Escoboza, Los Angeles County Department of Health; Mark Finucan, Los Angeles County Department of Health; Victor Freeman, Georgetown University Medical Center; Marsha Gold, Mathematica; William Gradison, Health Insurance Association of America; Dan Hawkins, National Association of Community Health Centers; Robert Hurley, Medical College of Virginia; Isadore King, The Wellness Plan; Sean O'Brien, Foundation Health Plan; Clyde Oden, United Health Plan; Lee Partridge, American Public Welfare Foundation; Anthony Rodgers, LA Care; Diane Rowland, Kaiser Family Foundation; Sara Rosenbaum, George Washington University, Center for Health Care Policy; and Patrick Williams, Georgia Department of Medical Assistance. We also appreciate the support that we received from the staff at the National Association of Public Hospitals & Health Systems, and the American Association of Health Plans for their assistance in formulating this book. Finally, we thank Liz Kramer for her editorial review and Ellen Derrick for her endless assistance in editing and producing this book.

The Authors

Dennis P. Andrulis is a health analyst with twenty-five years' experience on issues affecting vulnerable populations, their providers, and their communities. He has directed numerous projects and published extensively on these issues, including HIV hospital costs, urban social and health conditions, the role of the public sector in the era of managed care, and child health. He is also a founding member of the American International Health Alliance, which creates health partnerships between the United States and the nations of the former Soviet Union. Andrulis served as president of the National Public Health and Hospital Institute for ten years and is currently director of the Office of Urban Populations at the New York Academy of Medicine as well as adjunct professor at George Washington University. He holds a Ph.D. in educational psychology from the University of Texas at Austin and a master's in public health from the University of North Carolina at Chapel Hill.

Betsy Carrier has over twenty years of progressive management experience in health and health-related organizations. She has extensive experience in developing managed care plans and case management programs for individuals covered by both Medicaid and commercial insurance.

She is currently vice president for managed care at the National Association of Public Hospitals and Health Systems where she conducts education and training programs and provides consultation regarding all aspects of Medicaid managed care. She has an

MBA with a specialization in health care administration from the City University of New York and Mount Sinai School of Medicine. She lives in Bethesda, Maryland.

Introduction

This book is about the hope, promise, and uncertainty surrounding managed care in some of the most challenging environments in the United States, particularly in inner cities. It discusses community circumstances, financing, education, service providers, and many other facets affecting or related to managed care. But what truly lies at the heart of this book are the individuals whose well-being, if not lives, hang on the decisions and directions taken by the revolution in health care known as managed care.

Following are the stories of three hypothetical enrollees. Keisha, Rosa, and Jack are composite portraits drawn from sources as varied as policy reports and newspaper headlines on what the presence of managed care means for those who reside in inner cities. These stories set the tone for the rest of this book and personalize the importance of the dramatic changes that are occurring in health care, lending credence to why they demand the attention of policymakers, providers, and ordinary citizens alike.

Keisha

Keisha is a twenty-three-year-old single mother of two living in the inner city. After relying on public assistance for seven years, she found her first job, as a clerk in a small clothing store, thanks to her state's welfare-to-work program.

This transition has helped her move away from a cycle of dependence. However, it has also created unforeseen hardships.

Keisha does not know if she still qualifies for food stamps. The eligibility workers at the responsible city agency themselves do not seem to know, and as a result the application process has become more cumbersome. The state Medicaid program now says that she makes too much money to qualify for Medicaid managed care, and she must pay for her care herself. Her employer offered a plan with a minimum package of benefits, which she has joined, although it consumes a significant portion of her paycheck.

Her new managed care program is not the improvement over her Medicaid plan that she was led to expect. As with her previous Medicaid managed care program, providers under her current plan rarely maintain offices in her neighborhood. She has to travel with her children by bus for an hour to her new managed care physician, the second one she has had to choose in a year. She is used to having to change physicians in midyear; she also had to change physicians under her Medicaid program when he could no longer afford to see Medicaid patients. His capitation payments diminished as the state Medicaid program paid the managed care plan less, and the plan passed this reduction on to the providers.

With her new provider, Keisha waited two months before she could get a vision and hearing test for her son. But she does not think she can make the appointment since she has a full-time job and the doctor's office is not open on Saturdays. Of greater concern, however, is her daughter's asthma condition. Time and time again she has had to make the all-too-familiar trip to the emergency room when her daughter had an attack. Although the previous and current managed care plans approved her daughter's medication, their dusty, roach-infested apartment only leads to return visits to the emergency department. Keisha knows her daughter's condition will not improve over the long term until she makes changes in her home environment. The managed care plan pays only for medical care, however. Addressing Keisha's home needs directly or through education and public health, let alone participation in greater community health improvement efforts, are not part of the plan's scope of services.

Keisha is proud of her new job, but she is very worried that the health plan costs, and the continued difficulty of gaining access to care and services for her family, especially her daughter, is creating greater hardship. She is considering dropping her job and seeing if she can get back on welfare, or dropping her insurance and do what she used to do to stay healthy: pray and rely on the nearby public hospital emergency room.

Rosa

Rosa is a forty-two-year-old recent immigrant from Central America who came to the United States in 1995 and lives in a Latino section of a large city. She speaks no English and works sixty hours a week cleaning houses to support her teenage son and husband, a construction worker whose employment is seasonal; he has not had a job in three months.

The family has been uninsured since coming to the United States. Even though they could insure their son through the new state-federal child insurance program, they chose not to, for fear of being reported to the Immigration and Naturalization Service. Insurance payments are out of the question, given that virtually all of Rosa's income goes toward rent and food for her family and her sister, brother, and mother, who share their living space.

Rosa's few encounters with the health system to date have been difficult to negotiate. When her son's chronic diabetic condition required a trip to the emergency room, the local hospital had to ask a person from maintenance to translate, which he did with great difficulty since he did not understand the condition or the medical terminology. Rosa's use of alternative healers for her son—a familiar and well-used provider in her homeland—was ignored by the doctor and strongly discouraged by others at the hospital. Private providers in her area are rare: the deterioration of the neighborhood and the financial unattractiveness of the low-income residents have led most of the providers who practiced there to leave. With the exception of an overcrowded free clinic operated by the Catholic church, there are only a few remaining private urgent care centers—and they accept only cash.

A few months ago Rosa needed foot surgery. The bill was two thousand dollars. Her family temporarily lost a primary breadwinner and had to absorb a new, unanticipated debt. The safety net hospital that treated her has always maintained a mission to care for all regardless of ability to pay. But the pressures of managed care have placed greater pressure to minimize charity care and maximize revenues. As a result, it has adopted a more aggressive collection policy. The hospital now requires payment in full, although it agreed to a graduated plan to reimburse the hospital for Rosa's surgery.

As a result of the new costs, the troubling experiences with the health care system, and a perennial fear of trouble, if not deportation, occurring from any encounter with government-sponsored health care, Rosa and her family are likely to rely even more on lower-cost alternative healers and less on the health care system. Mother, father, and child are also likely to remain uninsured.

Jack

Jack is a sixty-one-year-old disabled individual who works at odd jobs. He had been covered by Medicaid fee-for-service until the state required that he enroll in the new Medicaid managed care program last year. His chronic condition requires a continuum of care and access to specialists. While he was covered under fee-for-service, he could gain access to specialty care fairly quickly; the new managed care program has restricted his access by requiring him to get a referral from his primary care gatekeeper. Now he must wait three times longer than before to get access to this care.

In addition to these problems, the deteriorating neighborhood has had its own negative effect on his health. His high blood pressure requires a careful diet, but there are only fast food franchises in his area; the local supermarket closed after a suspicious fire. The nearest pharmacy is fifteen blocks away. The violence and drug use in the area often make him a prisoner in his own apartment. And due to limits in his plan, there has been little room for home assistance since, according to the managed care program, he is not sufficiently disabled to qualify.

Recent copayment requirements have also greatly increased his prescription drug costs. He has begun to take some of his medication for his hypertension once every other day instead of daily as prescribed. Stretching out the doses also reduces his need to take the long trip to the drugstore.

Last month Jack received some bad news about his managed care plan. Unable to reconcile the costs of treating Medicaid enrollees with the dwindling financial coverage offered by the state, his plan sent notices to all members that it will cease offering coverage in six months. Given his already limited provider choices, he knows that the departure of his current plan after only a year or so does not bode well for future access to primary and specialty care.

Lost in the Maze of Managed Care

What these stories have in common is complexity. There is complexity, for example, in these individuals' home lives, in their professional lives, in their or their loved ones' health status, in gaining access to benefits, and in finding or keeping a doctor. Some of this complexity is coincidental. Managed care is not responsible for the emergence of welfare reform, the desertion by many stores and businesses of the inner city, shortcomings in transportation systems, the deterioration of inner-city schools, or the lack of social services for immigrants. To make a real difference, however, managed care must recognize and address such circumstances, which affect the health of individuals living in the inner city.

But perhaps more important, managed care is responsible for much of its own complexity, and it has yet to fulfill its guarantees of quality, access, affordability, and ease of use. This as-yet unrealized potential presents those concerned with health care in the inner city and elsewhere with a great opportunity. For when it works properly, managed care in both the private and public sectors has demonstrated it can be accountable for the quality of the services it provides, the value of the benefits purchasers obtain, and improvement in the health status of its enrollees.

This book is about helping those concerned with managed care and its responsibility to inner-city communities to understand, manage, and resolve the complexity. In so doing, managed care may yet fulfill its potential not only to provide medical care but to make a real difference in improving the health of those communities throughout the United States.

Managed Care and the Inner City

Chapter One

Managed Care and the Ecology of the Inner City

The term *inner city* conjures up many images. For some it brings to mind a difficult world with high rates of crime, deteriorated neighborhoods, and crowding. To others, however, these are places of commerce, where people work and live. They are also rich in culture and diversity. Indeed, there is no universally accepted definition of the inner city. For some, the phrase has come to be identified as a set of problems, when it more accurately should represent "an urban community as an integrated whole," with subpopulations, diversity, major problems, urban renewal, and related initiatives all a part of that whole (Koplan, 1993).

More than one in every five people in the United States lives in the one hundred largest cities, based on the 1990 census. Residents for miles around rely on health care delivered in those cities, which house some of the most prestigious medical facilities and most renowned doctors. As a result, the closing of a trauma center or burn unit in an urban area can have consequences that reach far beyond city limits. Furthermore, social changes in urban areas eventually reach less populated areas. One report (Wallace, Huang, Gould, and Wallace, forthcoming) strongly states that the "hyper-concentration" of violence, acquired immunodeficiency syndrome (AIDS), and related conditions is likely to diffuse out to suburban areas and smaller communities because of out-migration from inner cities and transportation links with outlying areas. As such, the challenges of the inner city have great relevance for managed care, health providers, and the United States generally.

This chapter discusses long-standing social and environmental circumstances, especially the influence of poverty and race, that frequently lead to poorer health among inner-city residents; and historical health care access problems of inner-city residents, in particular, a lack of mainstream insurance and imbalances in health practitioner supply within the inner city. The discussion highlights the myriad factors that significantly affect the organization, financing, and delivery of health services under managed care in the inner city.

The Inner-City Environment

Poverty and its impacts are primary causes of inner-city health concerns. The consequences of these factors, which have been called the "urban health penalty," were described at a New York Academy of Medicine meeting on the challenges facing health care in the nation's cities: when healthier, wealthier residents exit the city, they leave behind a larger proportion of minorities and sicker aged (Greenberg, 1991). The tax base shrinks, the physical environment deteriorates, businesses close or move, and abandoned buildings become homes to the homeless and the drug subculture. Police and fire departments neglect such areas, and they eventually burn or are otherwise destroyed. The cycle then begins at another site.

Survival in the Inner City

Manifestations of this penalty are widely evident. Residents of the inner city have access to fewer supermarkets, leading to lower levels of nutrition (Fossett and Perloff, 1995). At the same time, those in poor neighborhoods experience greater pressure to consume unhealthful products (exacerbated by cigarette and alcohol advertising in these neighborhoods). In some cases, poverty and poor nutrition combine to create an even more urgent and troubling situation (Nelson, Brown, and Lurie, 1998). A 1997 survey on hunger among over seven hundred interviewed adult patients at the public hospital in Minneapolis found that 12 percent reported insufficient amounts of food and 14 percent reported being hungry due to lack of money. Forty percent had used food stamps within the year.

Stress and depression are more prevalent among low-income populations (Parker, Greer, and Zuckerman, 1988). Daily living conditions can be so overwhelming to inner-city residents that simple survival can take precedence over what may be perceived as less immediate health concerns. Using focus groups of forty parents who were residents in Baltimore's inner city during 1990, a study found substantial resistance to participating in vaccination programs. Although the parents' groups were small, findings suggested that these inner-city residents perceived immunizations as a low priority, outweighed by perhaps more immediate and acute child health threats such as drugs and street violence (Keane and others, 1993). In addition, many inner-city residents have low-paying jobs that do not offer benefits. In these circumstances, staples such as food and housing often take priority over monthly health insurance premiums.

Housing and Homelessness

Deterioration of housing, a high incidence of fires, and overcrowding have been associated with increased incidence of numerous health conditions, including substance abuse, infant mortality, homicide, and various diseases, as well as greater need for hospital and emergency room care (Wallace, 1990).

Two reports on housing conditions in urban areas bring to light the depth and consequences of these problems. A 1997 study of living conditions in eight major inner-city areas (Bronx, East Harlem, St. Louis, Washington, D.C., Baltimore, Chicago, Cleveland, and Detroit) compared asthmatic children aged four to nine in neighborhoods where at least 30 percent of household incomes were below the poverty level (Rosenstreich and others, 1997). After reviewing health histories, the authors found that children who resided in inadequate housing were hospitalized 3.4 times more frequently than the others. An examination of lead toxicity among children in the Minneapolis area found that young enrollees at the HMO's urban clinics had blood lead levels three to eight times higher than those seen in the suburban clinics. (The HMO also found unexpectedly higher numbers of children with these elevated levels in suburban areas.) Age of the home was one of the most significant predictors of lead levels (Nordin, Rolnick, and Griffin, 1994).

Homelessness represents a real health danger. Premature death (in San Francisco the estimated average age of death among the homeless is forty-one years), AIDS, complications of alcohol, tuberculosis, pneumonia, and suicide all have been identified as health-related consequences of homelessness (Williams, 1991). A report based on over eighteen thousand admissions of homeless adults to public hospitals in New York City in the early 1990s found that over half were treated for substance abuse or mental illness and almost one-fifth were admitted for trauma, skin conditions, infectious diseases, and respiratory illnesses (Salit and others, 1998). Average lengths of stay were 36 percent longer per admission than other public hospital patients. The authors concluded that excess costs were associated with caring for this population.

Between 650,000 and 3 million people are estimated to be homeless at any one time in the United States. These individuals are more likely to live in cities. Recent estimates indicate that over 7 percent of the population (13.4 million) have been homeless at some time in their lives (Link and others, 1994).

Incidence of Disease

Table 1.1 describes the adverse effects of the urban health penalty as manifest by significantly greater rates of serious diseases. In the twenty-five largest U.S. cities in 1996:

- The tuberculosis rate was over twice the U.S. rate.
- Rates for syphilis were over three times the U.S. rate.
- Rates for AIDS were over one-third higher than the U.S. rate.

Nationally, infectious disease mortality increased 58 percent between 1980 and 1992, contrary to predictions, reports the Centers for Disease Control (Pinner and others, 1996), with the increase greatest in individuals aged twenty-five to forty-four years; human immunodeficiency virus (HIV) accounted for most of the increase. And although deaths due to AIDS have fallen dramatically in the past few years due to new drug treatments, the high number of individuals infected with HIV remains a great concern, both for stemming the tide of new cases as well as the annual costs related to treating those infected, which reaches $12,000 to $15,000 per year. There are other adverse consequences as well.

Substance Abuse. Alcohol and drug use remain entrenched problems. In 1991 26 million people reported using illicit drugs, 1.8 million were addicted to cocaine, and 700,000 were addicted to heroin. Five to 6 million were estimated to require drug treatment (Hamburg, 1993). Those who inject drugs rose from an estimated 50,000 in 1960 to 500,000 in the 1970s and 1.5 million in the mid-1980s (Musto, 1987). Substance abuse plays a contributing role in exacerbating other preexisting health conditions and is also a factor

Table 1.1. Selected Examples of the Urban Health Penalty: The Twenty-Five Largest Cities, 1996

Health Condition	City Incidence per 100,000	U.S. Incidence per 100,000	Percentage Difference
Tuberculosis	18	8	225
Syphilis	14	4	350
AIDS	30	22	36

Source: Andrulis and Goodman (1999). Used with permission.

in noncompliance with treatment. Cocaine use is linked with adverse health effects on the neonate, including low birthweight, prematurity, and small head circumference (Feldman, Minkoff, McCalla, and Salwen, 1992). This New York City hospital–based study examined pregnant women, and the authors concluded that cocaine contributes to the increased incidence of prematurity.

Alcohol consumption also contributes to congenital defects in neonates, ranging from fetal alcohol syndrome to increased risks of preterm delivery, reduced birthweight, and spontaneous abortions. A 1994 study found that black women are less likely to receive health behavior advice that could reduce their chances of having adverse pregnancy outcomes (Kogan, Kotelchuck, Alexander, and Johnson, 1994). Specifically, black women are less likely to report receiving smoking and alcohol cessation advice from their prenatal care advisers. There is a tendency for low-income and minority populations to have reduced access to care and to receive less thorough information related to healthy pregnancies.

Violence as a Public Health Threat. Notwithstanding recent pronouncements, overall, city residents still face a greater risk of exposure to violence: residents in cities fall victim to violence twice as often as others, according to a 1993 study of the one hundred largest U.S. cities (1,714 per 100,000 in cities; 803 per 100,000 for the United States) (Andrulis, Shaw-Taylor, Ginsberg, and Martin, 1995). Furthermore, in certain areas, the rate exceeded 3,000 per 100,000 in seven cities: Atlanta, Miami, St. Louis, Newark, Little Rock, Tampa, and Baton Rouge. Murder rates in cities in 1993 also were more than twice the U.S. average: 21 per 100,000 in the 100 largest cities versus 10 per 100,000 in the United States (Andrulis, Shaw-Taylor, Ginsberg, and Martin, 1995). And gang-related homicides—most prevalent in large cities but spreading to smaller cities—rose from 18 percent of the total killings in Los Angeles in 1979 to 43 percent in 1994 (Hutson and others, 1995). Inner-city residents tend to witness more violent behaviors in their homes and communities, which, the Centers for Disease Control (CDC) says, is a major contributor to repeated violent behavior. Research on violence has established a correlation between violence rates and community characteristics of socioeconomic status, including poverty, family structure and support systems, population density, community life, and the availability of firearms and drugs (Reiss and Roth, 1993).

The health consequences of violence extend far beyond criminal activity in many inner cities, and affect providers, families, and whole communities. A Philadelphia-based study of inner-city black women seen in hospital emergency rooms found that almost 40 percent sustained injuries that required care or resulted in death. Such injuries increased 55 percent between 1987 and 1990. Extrapolating from these findings, the authors suggest that violence affects women from this community in many aspects of their lives, extending far beyond the intimate heterosexual relationship (Grisso, Schwarz, Miles, and Holmes, 1996).

City hospitals treating victims of violence face great costs that their suburban counterparts do not encounter. Direct and indirect costs of gunshot trauma are $14.4 billion, with 86 percent of those costs borne by taxpayers. The hospital at the University of California at Davis (Kizer, Vasser, Harry, and Layton, 1995) reports that its average hospital charge for gun-related trauma between 1990 and 1992 was over $52,000. Resulting losses have been mainly offset by shifting these costs to those covered by private insurance.

Effects on Children and Youth. The challenges of the inner city often are most acute among its younger generation. Forty percent of urban children live below the poverty level (Andrulis, Shaw-Taylor, Ginsberg, and Martin, 1995). On any given night, an estimated 100,000 children have no place to live (Sabol, 1991). The National Center for Children in Poverty (1995) reports that the number of poor children under six years of age increased from 5 million in 1987 to 6 million in 1992. A study of 315 households with elementary school children in Hartford, Connecticut, found that over 41 percent experienced hunger in the previous twelve months and 35 percent experienced food shortages, placing them at risk for significant hunger (Singer, 1994).

Following are the major health consequences for children:

- Infant mortality is 60 percent greater for women with household incomes below the poverty level, and post-neonatal mortality is double the rate for women with household incomes above the poverty level (CDC, 1995).

- The rate of lead poisoning for poor children (household income under $6,000) is twice that in families with higher incomes (Agency for Toxic Substances and Disease Registry, 1988).

- Some 30 percent to 50 percent of city children are not immunized on time (Foltin, 1995).

- Suicide and homicide rates among children increased 200 to 300 percent between 1950 and 1993, but have risen especially since 1968. That increase more than offset decreases in conditions such as pneumonia, influenza, and cancer (Singh and Yu, 1996). These outcomes have been especially noticeable in the inner city. Most adversely affected are males and black, Native American, and Puerto Rican children.

- Between 1980 and 1988 the mortality rate for children in cities increased almost 50 percent, with firearms accounting for the increase, especially for young blacks (Koop and Lundberg, 1992).

- The infant mortality rate in the one hundred largest cities during 1989 was 12 per 1,000, 20 percent higher than the U.S. average of under 10 per 1,000 (Andrulis, Shaw-Taylor, Ginsberg, and Martin, 1995).

- Teenage birthrates followed a similar pattern, increasing in the one hundred largest cities at a rate far exceeding the 9.7 percent increase since 1980.

- Eighty-six percent of the victims of gang-related homicides in Los Angeles between 1979 and 1994 were between fifteen and thirty-four years of age (Ropp, Visintainer, Uman, and Treloar, 1995).

- Gunshot wounds have been the leading cause of death among black and white teenage boys in the United States (Koop and Lundberg, 1992).

- Minority children are most likely to be affected: A report on urban children (National Center for Children in Poverty, 1995) noted that over half of U.S. black and Latino children live in cities, versus only 25 percent of white children. Almost 40 percent of the children in New York City in 1987 were poor and, of them, 86 percent were African Americans. The American Medical Association's Council on Ethical and Judicial Affairs (1990) reports that health care for black Americans has improved since the 1960s; however, their infant mortality rate is twice the rate of the white population, and the decline in their mortality rate is lagging that of whites (Wise, 1992).

One frequently overlooked tragedy is the disproportionate incarceration of inner-city youth and young adults. Increases in the number of inner-city males who are in the penal or judicial system for criminal activity affect both family stability and concerns over safety in communities. Citing a number of studies, the New York Times reported in 1997 that cities are experiencing the consequences of dramatically increased numbers of younger black men being incarcerated. For example, half of Washington, D.C.'s black male population between eighteen and thirty-five years of age were in prison or jail or on probation. Such circumstances are likely to perpetuate inner-city crime due to connections between prison and the street. Long-term disruption to the family structure increases stress as well (Butterfield, 1997).

Access to the Health System

Social circumstances affect everyone regardless of heritage, undermining attempts to overcome what has come to be called "the urbanization of poverty" and its effects on health outcomes (Wilson, 1987).

Poverty, Death, and Disease

The consequences of this phenomenon are broad and deep. A 1991 article in the *Washington Post* based on a National Cancer Institute study of Atlanta, Detroit, and San Francisco highlighted that poverty had a much greater influence on cancer rates than did race or culture (Oakie, 1991). Individuals earning less than $9,000 annually in 1986 had death rates three to seven times higher (depending on race and gender) than those earning $25,000 or more (Fein, 1995).

At a given age, the death rate for people who do not graduate from high school is two to three times greater than those with college degrees (Fein, 1995). Only 23 percent of black males in the inner city graduate from high school, according to a report on urban violence after the riots related to the Rodney King police verdict in Los Angeles. Many are functionally illiterate, and unemployment among men ages nineteen to forty-five in the South-Central area reached 40 percent to 60 percent depending on the neighborhood (Shoemaker and others, 1993).

A comprehensive review of sociodemographic, health, and health behavior characteristics of over 300,000 white and 30,000 black men, using a baseline of 1973–1975 and running for sixteen years, confirmed a strong correlation between lower income and higher mortality regardless of race (Smith and others, 1996). Furthermore, it appears that the difference in health status because of income level may be increasing: reviews of British studies (Fein, 1995) found that in 1932, men in the lowest occupational group were 23 percent more likely to die prematurely than those in higher occupational groups. By 1970 that mortality difference had increased to 61 percent.

Finally, a longitudinal survey–based investigation on the interactions of education, income, and health behaviors on risk of death using over thirty-six hundred adult individuals supported the strong influence of socioeconomic factors (Lantz and others, 1998). In fact, the results indicated that while behaviors associated with low income contribute somewhat to an increased risk of dying, socioeconomic inequality is a stronger factor in predicting death, with the poor being exposed more often to occupational and environmental factors affecting their health, while lack of access may contribute to the deterioration of health.

Poverty and Violence

Poverty also makes it more likely a person will encounter violence. Studies in New Orleans and Atlanta found that a sixfold difference between black and white rates of domestic homicide was entirely accounted for by differences in socioeconomic status. Similarly, household crowding but not race was correlated with suicide rates (Centerwall, 1995).

A report by the Child Welfare League of America (Ards and Mincy, 1994) identified 880 disadvantaged neighborhoods in 1980 defined by having a high proportion of males over age sixteen not in the labor force, households headed by females, households on welfare, and high school–age dropouts. Ninety-nine percent of those neighborhoods were urban. They suffered high rates of child abuse, significant stress in the family, community instability, and a loss of social support networks.

Poverty and Family Effects

These circumstances account in large part for a 29 percent increase in foster care placements across the United States between 1986 and 1989. The consequences of such a breakdown in family and community are likely to show up in the health care system as higher rates of illness, greater emergency room use, and hospitalizations for avoidable conditions (Ards and Mincy, 1994).

Race and Ethnicity

Race and the economics and health consequences of poverty have become intimately linked in the cities. Over 40 percent of the black urban poor and 27 percent of Hispanic urban poor lived in high poverty areas in 1990 (Lawrence, 1994). This type of segregation has been identified as a predictor of age-standardized death rates for black urban residents aged fifteen to forty-four (Polednak, 1993). As Freeman (1993) points out, because racism and poverty create a strong interdependence that can influence who remains in poverty, providing health care access alone will not lead to improved health.

One in eleven (9 percent) blacks reported not receiving health care for economic reasons, whereas only 5 percent of whites reported such barriers. Black residents tend to live in states with the least generous Medicaid programs (the South and Southwest), and they are more likely to rely for health care on hospital clinics, community health centers, and related settings (Blendon, Aiken, Freeman, and Corey, 1989).

Certain diseases are more prevalent among blacks than whites. The life expectancy of African Americans in general is six years less than that of whites (Council on Ethical and Judicial Affairs, 1990). Men in Harlem in 1990 had a lower life expectancy than men in Bangladesh (McCord and Freeman, 1990). Infectious disease rates, which were 13 percent higher in African Americans than in the general population in 1980, were 36 percent higher by 1992 (Pinner and others, 1996). Blacks have a significantly higher incidence of nine cancers—lung, prostate, breast (under the age of forty), colon, pancreas, esophagus, cervix, stomach, and multiple myeloma—and the difference is increasing significantly. The rate of lung cancer is 45 percent greater in black men forty-five years old or younger than in their white counterparts (Clayton and Byrd, 1993). Black men are ten times more likely to die from hypertension than are white men (Lang and Polansky, 1994).

The number of asthma-related deaths among blacks rose from fewer than two thousand annually in 1978 to over forty-five hundred annually in the late 1980s—almost three times the white death rate for that condition (Lang and Polansky, 1994). Between 1985 and 1991, deaths in Philadelphia from asthma were significantly higher in census tracts with greater concentrations of blacks, Latinos, and persons below the poverty level (Lang and Polansky, 1994). Mortality from cirrhosis related to long-term heavy drinking is also greater for inner-city African Americans (CDC, 1995). By 1991 HIV had become the leading cause of death among blacks in the age group twenty-five to forty-four (National Center for Health Statistics, 1996).

Because of their concentration in inner cities, a higher proportion of blacks (37 percent) report use of illicit drugs at least once in their lifetime than whites (25 percent) (CDC, 1995). Latinos also face health challenges greater than other populations. The Latino poverty level, almost 29 percent, is only slightly less than the black rate (almost 33 percent) and substantially greater than the 14 percent for Asian–Pacific Islanders and less than 10 percent for white non-Latinos.

In a 1988 study (Mendoza, 1994), Latinos' risk of measles was three times greater than that of black children, and only 35 percent of Latino infants (12 percent of immigrant Latino children) were immunized by the age of two, compared with 47 percent for blacks. Hispanic youth have higher rates of cocaine use than other groups.

Latino women, 9 percent of the U.S. female population, represented almost 24 percent of reported AIDS cases among all women in the early 1990s. Twenty-four percent of childhood AIDS cases occur in the Latino population, even though they represent only 13 percent of U.S. children (Mendoza, 1994).

Since the 1970s, the homicide rate for Latino males in Los Angeles increased by almost 300 percent. By the late 1980s, Latino men were more than three and a half times more likely to die from homicide than other whites (Mendoza, 1994).

Poverty and the Effects on Quality of Care

Different perceptions on the part of both patients and caregivers play a role in access to health care. A mounting body of literature is demonstrating that programs attempting to address health care system inequities may need to recognize a complex interplay among physician practice patterns, institutional roles, patient income levels, and belief systems. In communities where people believe they have poor access to medical care, more patients are hospitalized for preventable chronic diseases such as asthma, hypertension, congestive heart failure, chronic obstructive pulmonary disease, and diabetes (Bindman and others, 1998). Blacks are less likely to be satisfied with their encounters with physicians, less satisfied with their hospital care, and more likely to believe their hospital stay is too short compared with white patients (Blendon, Aiken, Freeman, and Corey, 1989). Evidence suggests they may be right.

Kahn and others (1994) analyzed the quality of care in poor neighborhoods using duration of stay, instability in their condition at discharge, discharge destination, mortality, and medical processes for a multiyear sample of Medicare patients in the early to mid-1980s. They found that in urban hospitals, both nonteaching and teaching, patients who were black or from poor neighborhoods received worse processes of care and had greater instability than other patients.

A national survey of patients diagnosed with anterior myocardial infarction (Kahn and others, 1994) found that black men were only half as likely to undergo angiography and one-third as likely to undergo bypass surgery as white men, even though severity of illness was similar. A study of Massachusetts hospitals that controlled for income and severity also found racial patterns for coronary angiography, bypass, and angioplasty. The same is true in studies of dialysis and kidney transplants.

Other reports (Hayward, Shapiro, Freeman, and Corey, 1988) corroborate access problems for minorities, especially when compounded by poverty. Based on these findings, the American Medical Association's Council on Ethical and Judicial Affairs (1990) concludes that race plays an important role in medical care, and that income may influence medical decisions through the perception that greater wealth is equated with greater value to society. Other reports (Hayward, Shapiro, Freeman, and Corey, 1988) corroborate access problems for minority populations, especially those who are poor.

The Link to Insurance

Much has been written about the link between access and insurance. Although the consequences are often invisible for those who are insured, for the more than 40 million uninsured Americans, as well as those who are underinsured, this disposition affects both the care received and health outcomes, sometimes spelling the difference of outcome: health, disability, or death. A review of research and statistics highlights and confirms at least three well-established patterns: characteristics of the populations affected as measured by demographics and their ability to obtain services, compromises in receiving care, and the health effects related to lack of insurance.

Population Characteristics. The National Center for Health Statistics (1996) reports that black Americans were significantly more likely than white Americans to lack health insurance. Latinos were more than twice as likely not to have coverage as white persons. A survey of more than four thousand adults released by the Commonwealth Fund clearly portrayed the concerns of the urban poor in New York City (Sandman, Schoen, DesRoches, and Makonnen, 1998). According to their findings, for both New York City and the United States generally, the largest proportion of uninsured are in working families, with the vast majority near the poverty level.

The uninsured in New York City were more than twice as likely to report that they did not get the care they needed, compared to the insured population, and they were almost four times as likely to report difficulty in obtaining care (14 percent versus 53 percent for the uninsured). These patterns persisted when respondents were questioned about the availability of a regular physician and physician visits, as well as for specific services, such as mammograms or prostate exams for older adults. The uninsured also face more difficulty in paying medical bills. These and other access problems are more likely to affect populations of color. The locus of service for such populations is likely to be the emergency departments of public hospitals. Almost 50 percent of the uninsured in New York rely on these institutions for care.

Compromises in Receiving Care. In general, low-income populations receive fewer health care services compared with those who are more affluent. Although more services do not guarantee better health, there may be a threshold under which low-income populations are falling. *Health: United States, 1994* (National Center for Health Statistics, 1994) highlights the discrepancy between the poor (defined according to the U.S. Census as a family of four with an income below $16,036 in 1996) and the nonpoor. Between 1991 and 1993, nonpoor children under fifteen years of age received more ambulatory care than did poor or near-poor children. The average number of physician contacts per year for nonpoor children was 23 to 26 percent greater than for poor or near-poor children. Uninsured and underinsured inner-city populations may not be receiving the full range of services needed to treat their conditions adequately. For example, a 1994 report (NCHS, 1994) states that patients who visit office-based physicians are more likely to receive medication for asthma treatment and control and are more likely to return for repeat visits than those who visit the hospital only during acute attacks. Only 5 percent of the visits to office-based physicians do not include medication therapy; three times as many visits to the hospital do not include medication therapy.

Other reports document certain limits and obstructions to care. In a Boston study of fifty hospitals (Weissman and Epstein, 1989), uninsured patients received 7 percent fewer procedures and had 7 percent shorter hospital stays than patients covered by Blue Cross or Medicaid. These statistics imply that uninsured individuals receive less care even after hospitalization. A New York study (Burstin, Lipsitz, and Brennan, 1992) found that uninsured patients were at greater risk for substandard care associated with medical injury.

A survey of almost four thousand predominantly minority, disadvantaged patients presenting for ambulatory care during a seven-day period at a major public hospital in Atlanta found that lack of insurance and transportation, as well as having less than a high school education, were significant, independent predictors of delays and major obstacles to receiving care (Rask, Williams, Parker, and McNagny, 1994).

A self-reported survey of more than sixteen hundred individuals who used county clinics and emergency rooms in Seattle's King County found that the uninsured had the worst access, as determined by response to questions related to postponing care, denial of care, and the receipt of preventive services. Enrollment in Medicaid improved access, but not to parity with privately insured patients (Sayer and Peterfreund, 1993).

Even the presence of public insurance may not improve access. Research assistants posing as Medicaid patients in one study (Medicaid Access Study Group, 1994) called 953 urban ambulatory care clinics for appointments. The number of denials varied by location, but overall the study concluded that the Medicaid patients had significantly limited access to outpatient care beyond the emergency department.

Health Effects Related to the Lack of Insurance. It has been documented that being uninsured raises the risk of death across all sociodemographic and mortality groups, even after adjusting for gender, race, age, education, income, and documented employment. A report comparing uninsured and privately insured inpatients documented that virtually all groups lacking insurance had a higher relative probability of death in the hospital (Hadley, Steinburg, and Feder, 1991). A study that followed a group of patients over twenty-five years old for several years found that over 18 percent of the uninsured died compared with under 10 percent of the insured (Franks, Clancy, and Gold, 1993).

In all, the evidence is overwhelming that lack of mainstream insurance, and especially lack of any health insurance, significantly compromises access to care. Moreover, the numbers of uninsured are not likely to improve soon. In particular, the enormous changes in welfare reform leave great uncertainty about the ultimate impact on insurance status and access to health care. According to a 1997 article in the *Washington Post,* welfare assistance is the lowest since 1970, dropping almost 25 percent since 1992 (Harris and Havemann, 1997). One analysis suggests that the circumstances of cities with large numbers of working poor and immigrants may be similar to urban areas such as New York City, which witnessed an increase in the uninsurance rate among women under age eighteen from 14.4 percent to 19.4 percent between 1990 and 1995 (Fubani, 1997). The report further suggests that the number of uninsured people is likely to increase. Thus, the growing numbers in the inner city, especially poor and minority, may very well face disabling, if not life-threatening, consequences as a result.

Physician Supply Imbalance

The lack of physician availability for inner-city populations further encumbers their access and overall ability to obtain care. Several factors contribute to this difficulty: primary care physician shortages, distributions within these cities, and significant shortages of minority physicians.

Shortage of Primary Care Physicians. Cities have always attracted high concentrations of medical professionals. As Fossett and Perloff (1995) summarized, cities have three times as many general internists, four times as many pediatricians, and five times as many obstetricians/gynecologists as nonmetropolitan areas. These numbers, however, do not guarantee equal distribution of these professionals. Rather, distribution of these resources tends to follow higher incomes in the city or metropolitan area, thereby leaving serious shortages in the communities with greatest need. A review of city-specific studies (Fossett and Perloff, 1995) provides dramatic evidence of the shortage of doctors in inner-city neighborhoods—for example:

- In Chicago, there are 60 percent more children per pediatrician in the poorest areas than in the wealthiest areas.
- There are 6.4 doctors per 1,000 population in Manhattan but only 4 per 1,000 in the impoverished Bedford-Stuyvesant area of Brooklyn.
- There is 1 doctor per 125 residents of Beverly Hills but only 1 per 2,216 in the comparatively poorer El Monte community in the Los Angeles area.
- In Washington, D.C., the more affluent Northwest and related suburb of Bethesda, Maryland, have a pediatrician-to-child ratio of 1 to 400, contrasting with the poorer southeastern areas of the city, where the ratio is 1 to 3,700.

A second, more general factor adversely affecting health care in the inner city is the oversupply of specialists and the relative shortage of practitioners in primary care–related disciplines. It is generally accepted that access to and use of primary care services leads to better health. Shi (1992), for example, stated that access to a primary care provider was more strongly correlated with improved health than was number of hospital beds or specialty physicians.

Nonetheless, the high proportion of specialists has persisted, creating a significant gap that will take time to resolve. One projection (Politzer, Harris, Gaston, and Mullen, 1991) determined that the number of subspecialists was expected to increase more than 200 percent between 1978 and 1998, while the growth in general internists was expected to be only 77 percent. Over the 1980s, the level of interest in primary care–related specialties dropped from almost 39 percent to 25 percent. Family practice fill rates dropped from 85 percent in 1985 to 70 percent in 1990.

A number of factors contribute to this situation. One reason for this shortage is salary. In the early 1990s, for example, the average income for a family practitioner was $87,100, compared with an orthopedist's average income of $193,000. Another contributing factor is that teaching hospitals face financial disincentives to train primary care physicians. The revenue generated by residencies related to primary care services is significantly less than that of residencies oriented toward inpatient procedures. Family practice hospital-based residencies recover only 30 percent of their costs through patient care, compared with 81 percent of the costs of residency stipends generated in hospitals. Those differences are critical because institutions are relying more on service income (38 percent in 1987) than they did in the past (12.2 percent in 1970).

On a positive note, the national trend to specialization appears to be reversing. In 1989 only 11 percent of medical school graduates were planning careers in family practice (*Hospitals Magazine*, 1993). More recent reports on residency matching for postgraduate medical training indicate sharp shifts toward more primary care–oriented areas. In fact, a majority of recent medical school graduates are choosing primary care programs such as internal medicine, pediatrics, and family practice (Association of American Medical Colleges, 1996).

Within-City Distribution Problems. Vulnerable populations in the inner city may not benefit from increasing numbers of primary care specialists because inner cities are unattractive locations for physicians (Fossett and Perloff, 1995). Major disincentives include lower numbers of individuals with disposable income, unpleasant social conditions (drug abuse, violence, poverty), a sicker population, language differences, higher rates of noncompliance and missed appointments, limited ability of the medical care system to affect factors in the patient's environment such as homelessness and crime, and the perception that malpractice suits are more likely to occur in such areas.

Inner-city finances remain an obvious hurdle. The growing number of poor households concentrated in very depressed inner-city areas and their reliance on Medicaid make it difficult to offset lower reimbursement with privately insured patients ("Low Medicaid Fees . . . ," 1991). Medicaid pays doctors only 69 percent of the private insurance rate, according to a Physician Payment Review Commission study. That is a major reason that forty-four states have difficulty in soliciting doctors to participate in Medicaid.

Even doctors who do practice in cities tend to gravitate to areas with higher incomes, while many inner-city residents live in areas that are underserved. There was a 45 percent decline in office-based primary care physicians in ten urban areas between 1963 and 1980 (Kindig and others, 1987). The number of Health Professional Shortage Areas designated by the federal government declined 9 percent from 1985 to 1988, but then rose 2 percent by 1990. According to the Bureau of Primary Health Care, half of those populations are in urban areas (U.S. Department of Health and Human Services, 1993a).

In all, although the total number of physicians has increased over the past twenty-five years, evidence strongly indicates this growth has done little to reduce the shortage of physicians providing care for inner-city residents. More recent competitive pressures may alter this situation by making previously less attractive populations and locations more desirable for health care providers. However, the temptation to be selective in inner-city settings may significantly offset the potentially positive impact.

Shortage of Minority Physicians. A final critical issue is the shortage of minority physicians overall and a dearth of doctors in minority communities. Reports on physician availability (*Hospitals and Health Networks*, 1996) have documented a connection with race and ethnicity. A 1996 study in California (Komaromy and others, 1996) reported the lowest proportion of doctors-to-population in poor urban communities with high proportions of black and Hispanic residents. In contrast, poor urban areas with low proportions of those populations had three times as many primary care physicians. Similar patterns were found for rural areas.

Medical school enrollment of minorities has lagged the growth of those populations: minority populations grew 18.5 percent between 1975 and 1990, but minority medical school enrollment rose only 7 percent (Rivo and Satcher, 1993). As a result of these trends, responsibility for health care services that people in the inner city need frequently falls to a few providers willing to treat patients with little money and many, and often complex, problems. These trends also identify why a number of inner-city communities are so dependent on international medicine graduates who may be more willing to serve in such health care settings. In general, foreign medical school graduates were more likely to practice in these areas than U.S. medical graduates. Left unaddressed, initiatives eliminating affirmative action in California and elsewhere will only worsen this situation by reducing the already limited pool of minority physicians willing to care for minority populations.

Conclusion

The quality and characteristics of communities where people live and work clearly affect their health in significant ways. Inner cities, however, present their own array of additional factors that influence or even determine the health of populations. Managed care organizations and providers must consider these determinants in their organization and delivery of services:

- Community and population issues such as housing, concentrations of poverty, crime, and basic priorities related to survival that can take precedence over health care
- Cultural diversity in these settings that requires knowledge of patterns and history of disease, as well as how to provide health care tailored to the specific needs of given populations

- Disease-specific challenges such as HIV/AIDS, violence-related injuries, substance abuse, tuberculosis, and aggravating conditions such as homelessness
- Special access challenges such as concentrations of those without insurance, inadequate provider distribution, and quality or continuity of care limitations and lack of minority health practitioners

If managed care and the related provider networks as well as the sources of support are able to structure their system to lessen the urban health penalty, then they may achieve true progress in improving the health of inner-city residents. Left unaddressed by key participants and a policy of neglect, these factors will bankrupt those who do try but are insufficiently capitalized, perpetuate already chronic underservice, and leave residents possibly worse off, especially if the traditional health care safety net is undermined by a turbulent marketplace.

Chapter Two

Managed Care, the Safety Net, and Inner-City Residents

By 1996 more than 58 million people were enrolled in HMOs, and another 91 million were receiving services through managed care arrangements (Halverson and others, 1997). According to the Health Care Financing Administration, as of June 1997, over 15 million people were enrolled in Medicaid managed care. With this accelerated expansion come questions about whether managed care can provide high-quality care to vulnerable populations and whether organizations that traditionally have treated these populations, most notably public health, public hospitals, and community health centers, can sustain their well-established mission.

Managed Care Organizations: Benefits and Concerns for the Inner City

Managed care is not new to the inner city. In fact, for some urban communities such as New York City and many California cities, the current emphasis is an evolutionary step. Nevertheless, the potential benefits of expanded managed care to inner-city communities are great: creating a comprehensive network of care; successful continuity of care; increased access, especially to primary care; more efficient, cost-effective use of resources; and using nonphysician providers to improve access to primary care in particular. As in other settings, imposing a network model in the historical context of a fragmented set of services in the inner city could yield great benefits for these communities.

Individuals enrolled in Medicaid can benefit from managed care if plans help patients make informed choices about their care. Ideally patients enrolled in managed care plans have access to credentialed providers who have incentives to focus on prevention and health education. Managed care theoretically improves continuity of care and reduces fragmentation of services. In a fee-for-service environment, it has become increasingly difficult for Medicaid patients to obtain specialty care because Medicaid fee-for-service payment schedules in some states are so low that recipients often cannot find a physician who will accept Medicaid. Medicaid managed care can improve access by often providing patients with a medical home and needed specialty care.

Managed care creates a contractual obligation to provide services at a designated place. When it is well administered, providers who practice in a managed care setting can improve the coordination of care and are more attentive to the needs of patients. Managed care is also better organized to teach enrollees about prevention as well as treatment. Managed care plans have a greater incentive than fee-for-service providers to develop and implement quality and practice standards, as well as effective information systems.

Notwithstanding these potential benefits, concerns have arisen about the application of managed care principles for vulnerable populations in urban settings.

Illness, Poverty, and Outcomes in Urban Settings

A number of studies conducted in the 1990s focused on managed care access and quality for vulnerable, impoverished populations. One project followed 2,235 chronically ill elderly and poor (living at or below 200 percent of poverty-level income—frequently defined as "near-poor") patients in three urban areas (Los Angeles, Chicago, and Boston) for four years, comparing fee-for-service and HMO-based providers as part of the ongoing Medical Outcomes Study (Ware and others, 1996). Their report documented that elderly HMO patients had poorer health outcomes than those in fee-for-service settings. Those in poverty tended to experience a greater decrease in health status. The authors noted that the HMO patients cited fewer financial barriers and more effective service coordination, but the fee-for-service patients experienced shorter waits, more comprehensive care, and better continuity of care, as well as a higher rating of quality of care. In all, the elderly and poor were more than twice as likely to suffer declines in health status in the HMO setting (individuals who were younger, in relatively good health, and relatively well off fared better in HMOs). Medicaid coverage for the poor did not explain the difference.

A survey-based review of low-income adults in five states reinforced these concerns. It found that the adult Medicaid population was poorer and sicker than a privately insured group. The authors concluded that private managed care plans may need to adjust their organization, in particular their health care delivery and administrative approaches, if they are to serve a Medicaid enrollee population. Moreover, Medicaid beneficiaries cited more problems in locating providers who will see them (Lillie-Blanton and Lyons, 1998).

Access to and Quality of Care for Women and Children

In 1989 Pennsylvania implemented a Medicaid managed care demonstration project that included case management and initiatives to address broader community health concerns in two low-income neighborhoods in Philadelphia (Henley and Clifford, 1993). One of the managed care plans served eighty-two thousand predominantly minority enrollees.

The U. S. General Accounting Office assessment (1993) of the program cited numerous shortcomings. It found that regardless of level of care received, the low-income women had high rates of prematurity and low-birthweight babies. Moreover, many children enrolled in this program were not receiving federally mandated screening and preventive care services. The program, HealthPASS, also had little success in enrolling more women for Women, Infants, and Children (WIC) services. The assessment documented ineffective utilization management as more services were provided and reimbursement levels were increased. The report concluded that offering Medicaid managed care to this population did not necessarily increase either the amount or the quality of health care received, and the outreach programs did little to increase enrollment in federal aid programs.

Another study investigated the shift of more than 1 million Los Angeles Medicaid beneficiaries into mandatory managed care. This transition has been far from smooth (American Medical Association, 1997). LA Care Health Plan was expected to be the largest plan, but federal officials halted enrollment just two weeks after the enrollment period was launched. The Health Care Financing Administration (HCFA) criticized the plan for having done too little to orient beneficiaries to the new system and for limiting patient choice by delays in plan start-up. The problems were confounded by the fact that many of the people affected by the changes did not speak English, and they reported having discarded the enrollment materials the county sent out because the materials were too complex. Of the initial 100,000 beneficiaries, 60 percent did not select a plan. Due to implementation difficulties, as of 1997 there were many unassigned beneficiaries in fee-for-service. Meanwhile, the managed care plans have been attempting to satisfy new state record-keeping requirements. In meeting these requirements, some plans have administrative costs that are as much as 30 percent of the premium.

These reports raise two important questions. Do these events represent examples of start-up problems in difficult inner-city markets? Or do they represent deeper structural problems in broad-based application of managed care? Concerns related to the first question might be resolved through initially slower or smaller-scale transition to managed care. The second question, however, suggests the need for a more exacting review of the program's capacity to address the needs of inner-city populations.

Scope of Health-Related Services for Vulnerable Populations

Substantial numbers of inner-city residents suffer from chronic conditions that are aggravated by exposure to poor living conditions and health system neglect. One study documented that inner-city children covered by Medicaid have a higher incidence of chronic and debilitating conditions than do their privately insured counterparts (McManus and Fox, 1996). There is a dramatic disparity in service use between these two populations. The need for more preventive services, more physician visits, and more support services for children with chronic conditions is proving a struggle for HMOs. McManus and Fox suggest that HMOs alter their services to provide for this population. Changes include specially trained primary care physicians, improved screening and risk assessment, diagnosis and evaluation teams, health education, flexible gatekeeping arrangements, and coordination with public health, education, and social services.

In addition to the concerns over children enrolled in managed care plans, there are high costs attendant to many chronic illnesses and related concerns for low-income Medicare beneficiaries with chronic illnesses who are enrolled in health plans (Fox and Fama, 1996). Issues that surface include selection bias, addressing fears of people with chronic conditions who are required to join managed care plans, and quality of care. To meet patient needs, HMOs must analyze the populations they serve, begin disease-specific programs, and improve services to reduce the difference between current practices and best practices and improve case management for patients with chronic illnesses. To achieve these goals, plans need longitudinal data tracking to monitor functional status, case management, and strengthened utilization review that focuses more on chronic care. One report straightforwardly warns that if managed care organizations lack sufficient funding and case managers, they will have a difficult time succeeding in this arena (McGuire, 1996).

Cultural Challenges

Many health plans will need to reorient their programs to care for populations from many cultures who bring their own beliefs about health care. Health plans must incorporate their served populations' cultural beliefs in order to treat patients effectively. In addition, language translation capacity becomes central to many health care transactions. In an era where English is the second language to as many as 32 million people in the United States (13 percent of the U.S. population according to the 1990 U.S. Census), many of whom reside in cities, competence in interpretation and cultural issues is rapidly becoming an essential capability for health care providers. Meeting these needs, however, may be very difficult given the frequent focus on the near-term bottom line and the failure by some to see the tangible monetary payoff of such efforts.

Image of Managed Care Among Inner-City Residents

Finally, historical and environmental issues may have created suspicions regarding the motivation of managed care organizations that operate in inner cities. In particular, mistrust of these organizations by the inner-city population may be built around experiences in which certain cities were havens for unfair marketing practices. In certain markets plans may take advantage of individuals through questionable marketing practices, for example, advertising in a language to attract individuals but having very few practitioners familiar with that culture or any language facility. In some cases, enrollees in these markets never receive adequate services. As a result, inner-city communities have become skeptical about the motivation of outside plans. This has led to a commercial image problem that can impede success in both the market and member care. Some private managed care organizations that are not well established in inner cities may have little experience with these populations. For them, their unfamiliarity may lead to significant adverse economic and patient care outcomes.

Managed Care Responses to Inner-City Populations and Their Health Care Needs

Many health plans have adopted innovative strategies to address the special circumstances of inner-city residents, especially as they choose to focus on Medicaid and similar programs for the working poor. The following are selected examples of such initiatives.

Broad Education and Community Initiatives

HMOs are using videos, orientation sessions, telephone support, and other ways to educate enrollees about their plans (Politzer, 1995). These communication options describe services available to enrollees, inform enrollees of how to negotiate the system, and answer common questions. Henry Ford Health System in Detroit, Harvard Pilgrim Health Plan in Boston, and other health plans have applied information system expertise to track and review patient care and the health of the community (Showstack and others, 1996).

One approach to address these issues, undertaken by Foundation Health in Los Angeles, was to create a consumer advisory committee and community liaison group. While clearly intending to improve marketing, its objectives also include identifying community needs and considering collaboration with other key informal organizations. As part of this initiative, Foundation Health employed forty individuals for community outreach.

Health Care Services Extending into the Community

Certain managed care organizations have explicitly pursued activities that affect both their enrollees and the community at large. For example, the Health Insurance Plan (HIP), an HMO in New York City, with long-standing experience in urban areas, has offered free immunizations to several thousand preschool children, both plan members and nonmembers ("HIP to Offer Free Childhood Immunizations," 1993).

Bronx Health Plan, Bronx, New York
Interview with Maura Bluestone, Executive Director

The Bronx Health Plan (TBHP) began operations in 1987 as a non-profit prepaid health plan licensed in New York State under the HMO Licensing Authority. It serves Medicaid and an uninsured population through a network model where community physicians practice from their offices. TBHP is a network model plan, with most primary care provided by physicians who practice in community health centers.

In its early years, TBHP was able to expand services, invest in primary care capacity development, and still be financially successful with capitated premium payments. However, dramatic declines in premium rates, coupled with a larger benefits package and higher administrative and reporting requirements, led to financial losses in 1996 and 1997. In 1996 every health plan in New York City that served Medicaid patients lost money.

TBHP believes that for managed care to be effective, it must assume responsibility for service delivery while ensuring quality of care. It believes that when managed care is implemented and used properly, it can lead to an effective use of dollars, rationalize service delivery, and have built-in accountabilities. Managed care can provide an appropriate and responsive network for the inner city by offering or helping to coordinate a wide range of social and welfare support services.

To succeed, TBHP found it needed to work with other agencies. Coordinating all of the services is necessary so that the delivery system does not become increasingly fragmented. For example, TBHP finds that it needs to offer and coordinate translation and transportation services. Most of the staff is bilingual in English and Spanish, and they also work with AT&T's language banks, wherein a health professional can call an available number and be connected with a translator.

Private networks need public suppliers because they may be either the major or only provider of care in certain areas. Often it has been in the plan's best interest to have contractual relationships with these public providers. However, it has been difficult to establish and make these relationships successful.

Given the marketplace changes in New York City, there is no clear vision for the future of Medicaid managed care. TBHP is dedicated to serving low- and moderate-income urban populations. It seeks to improve its service delivery to public clients. To do this, it must grow, achieve economies of scale in administration, and leverage costs when buying services. However, shrinking state Medicaid rolls are reducing revenues. Perhaps of greater concern is the reduction in state rates that has led to the loss of critical support used to finance indigent care and capital efforts. Together with the potential loss of community health under involvement due to buyouts from hospitals, and their reluctance to participate due to insufficient reimbursement, TBHP faces great difficulty in maintaining its network.

Targeted Disease Interventions

In recognition of the concentration of certain conditions among many urban residents, a number of managed care plans have directly targeted specific communities with the objective of reducing those conditions or alleviating adverse affects while lowering health care costs. Harvard Pilgrim Health Plan recognized the high cost and high morbidity associated with asthma, a typical inner-city health problem, and established the Asthma Outreach Program, the Central Pediatric Asthma Program, and a physician education program (Greineder, 1996). These initiatives have demonstrated some success in decreasing emergency room use, hospitalization, and high use of resources for this condition.

Lovelace Health Systems in Albuquerque, New Mexico, has instituted a new program, Episodes of Care (EOC), which is similar to disease management. The program focuses on clinical practice data-driven decisions (Friedman, 1997b). Lovelace has implemented EOCs for diabetes, pediatric asthma, coronary artery disease, pregnancy and childbirth, low back pain, breast cancer, stroke, depression, and knee care. The EOC team includes specialists and primary care physicians, nurse case managers, health educators, quality measurement specialists, clinicians, physicians and mid-level practitioners (for example, family nurse practitioners), pharmacists, and support personnel with relevant knowledge. In this community, researchers have noted a difference in hospitalization rates between the managed care population and the fee-for-service population, which lacked this comprehensive educational program.

Plans also have come to recognize that caring for Medicaid patients with AIDS-related pneumocystis carinii pneumonia (PCP) in a prepaid, multidisciplinary, coordinated care system has several benefits. The Community Medical Alliance (CMA) contracts with Massachusetts Medicaid on a fully capitated basis to provide a comprehensive set of benefits to the medically complex cases of pneumocystis. An evaluation compares the findings of the CMA population to a New York population on the incidence of PCP episodes, location of care, and treatment outcomes. The benefits CMA provides include reduced barriers to care through the use of nurse practitioners, thereby lowering the incidence and stage of pneumocystis through home care (Master 1996).

Safety Net Providers, Managed Care, and Vulnerable Populations

Public hospitals, health centers and clinics, and health departments that comprise a large component of what has come to be called the health safety net in many urban areas are experienced in caring for residents of the inner city. This experience can benefit both patients and providers in the evolution of managed care in the inner city. The following narrative identifies key inner-city provider issues involving the safety net. Their described role in addressing these issues may provide direction for managed care and related Medicaid or other low-income programs.

Safety Net Provider Location

Clearly not all commercially sponsored managed care plans are unfamiliar with the populations who reside in the inner city. However, for those that may not be prepared for the service needs and the characteristics of the enrollee group, safety net providers may serve as important allies. A report (GHAA and KPMG, 1994) on the relationship of seven, primarily urban-based HMOs to vulnerable populations and safety net providers indicated that in certain inner-city areas, safety net, or "essential community," providers tend to be more concentrated in underserved areas than the traditional private HMO provider. As such, contracting with essential community providers in caring for the indigent may represent an increasingly attractive option for plans.

Service for Difficult-to-Treat Patients

Safety net providers may be one of the only groups willing to provide services for difficult-to-treat individuals. For example, a medical record review of homeless and low-income individuals studied whether the homeless had reached health parity with their housed counterparts through their use of a major community ambulatory health center in West Los Angeles (Gelberg, Doblin, and Leake, 1996). Findings documented that homeless patients received more procedures and services than domiciled patients did. The homeless also received atypical managed care services, such as showers, travel vouchers, and advocacy. These services may be crucial to ensure patient trust and motivation to seek medical care and compliance with follow-up care.

Community Involvement

In other cases, participation by the urban community is a critical step in diagnosing, educating, and managing the care of vulnerable populations. A demonstration project sponsored by the American

Cancer Society established a comprehensive cancer prevention, education, and diagnostic clinic in an inner-city West Oakland, California, community (Renneker and others, 1994). Between 1989 and 1992 the clinic served 2,058 patients, of whom nearly 50 percent were uninsured. Their screening uncovered twenty-two precancers and fifteen cancers, and their clients demonstrated significant gains in knowledge, improved attitudes, and nutritional and lifestyle behavior. In addition to the clinic service activities, the education program reached almost fifteen thousand community residents. The evaluation found this intervention successful at reaching indigent inner-city residents. Project assessment concluded that the indigent will use cancer prevention if it is made available and conducted in their community.

Adaptability to Population Needs

The Watts Health Foundation (WHF), with its HMO United Health Plan (UHP), has focused its efforts on inner-city vulnerable populations (Oden, 1994). It serves an estimated 125,000 individuals and provides more than 250,000 encounters per year. Among other activities, its focus is on addressing access by locating services and facilities in the neediest neighborhoods. Services include mobile medical centers, schools, social agencies, churches, and local parks and using health providers from the National Health Services Corps. An objective of WHF is to improve outcomes of certain conditions, such as high levels of sexually transmitted diseases and low levels of childhood immunizations. It accepts the responsibility for improving the health status of its members, including becoming an active participant and an advocate for improving the community's health. As such, the foundation extends its efforts to include health education on sexually transmitted diseases, nutrition and WIC programs, and substance abuse prevention and treatment. In the context of community reinvestment, it also encourages working with the business sector and has established an affiliated bank that assists in providing low-interest loans.

Some promising results have been documented from UHP's efforts. For example, its Healthy Black Babies program reduced the infant mortality rate from twenty to sixteen per thousand in a group of primarily Medicaid enrollees (Harris and others, 1996). It also successfully worked through the WIC program to increase breastfeeding. Another California program, LA Care, the public managed care program for Los Angeles, stresses member and community health. LA Care incorporates linguistic and cultural competence formats to meet the diverse needs of its enrollees. The focus is on enrollee education, and it reaches beyond traditional member handbooks by distributing audiotapes to enrollees and community members. Efforts to reach and educate residents include creating support groups for adolescent mothers, peer groups, and providing incentives such as food coupons, diapers, and movie tickets in an attempt to change negative behaviors. In this example, a safety net managed care organization has involved nontraditional participants such as grocery stores, theaters, and other organizations using plan enrollees as a potential future customer base.

United Health Plan, Los Angeles, California
Interview with Clyde Oden, president

Founded in 1973, UHP, with 1997 revenues of $200 million and 820 employees, is the largest community-based health organization in the United States. It also is one of the first community-based organizations to have developed a managed care contract. UHP owns and operates a varied range of products: a managed care plan, two federally qualified health centers (FQHCs), two substance abuse clinics, a school-based clinic, thirteen mobile vans, health education programs, and various subcontracts. Services are made available to residents of the Los Angeles inner city.

As part of the California Medicaid two-plan model, the state contracts with a publicly sponsored plan and a private sector plan. This model offers the recipient a plan choice. UHP operates as the private sector plan in Los Angeles. The plan has been successful as a Medicaid plan; however, recently it has suffered from the vagaries of decision making regarding the roll-out of Medi-Cal, the California Medicaid managed care program. The most recent problem has been the delay in implementing guidelines for how Medicaid enrollees are handled when they do not select a plan. The delays for developing default plan guidelines have cost UHP an estimated $25 million in lost revenues, resulting in the plan's having to lay off staff. In addition, the state does not want to pay United Health Plan FQHC rates, which would result in an additional $7 million loss.

One of the key consequences of the loss of support to the plan is that service to the indigent is severely compromised. UHP estimates that the indigent care caseload in 1996–1997 was reduced 30 percent from the previous year. In addition, immigrants' fear of deportation or being reported to the INS has caused many Hispanic patients not to seek needed care.

Strategies for survival have included participating in various business coalitions. Over time UHP has adapted by becoming a community service enterprise and a nonprofit holding company that has for-profit and nonprofit spinoffs that operate health care programs, social services, and a bank that returns support to the community through home loans.

UHP has been instrumental in starting the Urban HMO Coalition, which comprises managed care organizations that have 50 percent or more low-income enrollees, are located in major urban areas, are for profit and nonprofit, and are predominantly minority based.

UHP believes that federal policy should develop requirements to monitor how managed care affects the health of the vulnerable populations. In monitoring plans, it will be difficult to make comparisons across payer classes because of the basic differences in the design of Medicaid and commercial managed care programs. Clyde Oden believes there is a fundamental question as to whether the public sector can truly be regulator, purchaser, and provider.

Managed Care, the Safety Net, and the Need to Become Part of the Community

Finally, managed care must recognize that the nonmedical safety net plays a critical role in caring for vulnerable inner-city populations and serving as a bridge to the health system. When literacy and language present challenges, there may be an increased need to draw on community resources such as churches and community centers for health education and outreach. Moreover, since violence and drugs play such influential roles in the inner city, coordination with youth centers, the police, and government agencies may be essential. As a result, in many urban areas managed care will need to consider integrating this informal safety net as part of more comprehensive initiatives to develop and improve the health of their enrollees and their community. These directions may run counter to the traditional managed care organization's functions as a closed system within which enrollees and service providers alike are either "in or out." In the effort to address the needs of inner-city residents, the broader ecology, including a mix of social challenges, language differences, entrenched poverty, deteriorating housing and streets, violence, nutrition, and many other factors, will need to be seriously considered as integral to many interventions.

Conclusion

By its design and intended effect, managed care represents a potentially substantial advance in organizing and delivering services in the inner city. It presents an opportunity for providers to offer an effective continuum and spectrum of critical services. Historically those who live in these areas have faced fragmented, discontinuous care that frequently is delivered through hospital outpatient clinics and emergency departments. However, evidence to date on managed care's progress in resolving these problems is at best mixed.

Although no organized national trend is evident to create broad-based strategies to inner-city vulnerable populations, individual managed care plans have developed initiatives to address health and health-related conditions. These include enrollee education and tracking of patient care needs, offering services such as immunizations to the community at large, and more comprehensive interventions to manage the care of HIV patients and others with special needs. The question remains as to whether these will remain isolated instances or whether managed care plans will make them part of a more systematic approach to addressing the needs of the inner city.

Finally, providers that constitute the urban safety net have extensive experience with inner-city populations. This experience can inure to the benefit of managed care organizations as well as provide a firm base for plans developed by safety net providers. These experiences include convenient and established locations of services in urban areas; familiarity with caring for patients from diverse racial and ethnic backgrounds; concentration in underserved areas; flexibility in adapting to population needs and working with other safety net providers such as public health; knowledge of the broad range of services, both health and health related, required by many inner-city residents; extended relationships to a broad spectrum of key organizations such as the police, youth centers, and social service programs; and collaboration and integration with the community, including serving as an advocate for community needs. A key unanswered question is to what extent many of these strengths will be seen as core to the mission of managed care.

Chapter Three

Implementing Managed Care
in the Inner City

As managed care becomes a vehicle for providing services in urban areas, questions arise as to how managed care organizations that are entering into or expanding in cities will take advantage of new opportunities, and how they will interact with practitioners such as public and private clinics and hospitals, physicians, and health departments that historically have provided care to inner-city residents. These new organizations will develop a wide range of relationships with existing providers, from competitors to collaborators.

Corporate missions will play a key role in these decisions. Managed care organizations include both for-profit and not-for-profit organizations that either have service delivery track records or have been created exclusively to take advantage of real and perceived profit-earning opportunities. Corporate-level contracting decisions and a willingness to serve certain populations will have profound effects on the scope and composition of managed care relationships. *Managed Community Health: An Integrated Model,* by the Archbishop's Commission on Community Health in St. Louis (Gales, 1996), addressed these complexities. This publication stressed the need to move health resources to places where people spend most of their time, for example, the home, the workplace, places of worship, and schools. Implementation of health care services also should focus on using preestablished community resources.

This chapter identifies organizational issues that managed care plans and providers face as they apply managed care principles and objectives to the inner city. For traditional providers of care to urban vulnerable populations, including those developing their own plans, it also discusses the additional challenges they face in incorporating managed care into their mission, management, and operations.

Community Health and Public Health Issues

The expansion of managed care's influence raises uncertainties about the fit of many responsibilities within its original objectives of continuous and cost-contained health care. Community health and public health are key examples of such responsibilities and the ambiguity surrounding what role, if any, that managed care will adopt.

Local health departments represent a key service sector that is caught up in these circumstances. These departments traditionally have assumed responsibility for providing direct individual health care and monitoring and surveillance services within their communities. Among their general activities are evaluating health status and needs, keeping track of communicable diseases, developing policies to fit their communities, and providing immunizations, family planning, and well-child care. Seventy-five percent of the resources used to support local health departments were devoted to primary care and communicable disease programs, with environmental health and administrative activities accounting for most of the remaining support (Studnicki and others, 1994). These services have been a mainstay for the working poor and indigent; in Kentucky, in 1993, for example, 65 percent of respondents on a telephone survey used health departments for childhood immunizations because of their financial circumstances.

This pattern is changing with the advent of managed care, however. In a recent survey of 176 local health departments in areas with over 100,000 population (Peck and Hubbert, 1994), only 56 percent reported that they continue to provide direct primary and preventive health care services, including immunizations and family planning. A number were questioning whether their departments should continue to provide such services or whether their role might be better focused on prevention, education, and health promotion. Indeed, many are switching to nonclinical activities, especially outreach, health education, and strengthening provider linkages.

But local health departments expressed concerns about managed care, particularly concerning substantial or even drastic reduction in services, clients, and related revenues (up to an 80 percent decrease in child health visits due to erosion of patients); fear they would have insufficient capitation rates; inability to provide services to high-risk populations (in some cases, clients were turned away from immunization and lead screening due to lack of reimbursement); a focus on only medically necessary care, reducing nutrition, prevention, and related services; the virtual elimination of early and periodic screening, diagnosis, and treatment programs in many locales; and the need for staff retraining to adapt to managed care and downsizing. Recognizing the increased competition and cost reductions, several noted concern that the burden on cities and counties to care for low-income, uninsured, and undocumented persons could increase as private sector managed care programs severely restrict the ability to shift costs to other sources.

A 1996 Centers for Disease Control (CDC) meeting brought together public health agencies and HMOs and stressed the value each brings to improving prevention and primary care (Harris and others, 1996). Among its conclusions were these:

- HMOs have the opportunity to participate actively in promoting community health.
- Public health agencies could reconsider their roles in the context of a reorganized health system.
- Public health departments bring key experience in surveillance, information systems, applying policy for public health purposes, case management, and access improvement for vulnerable populations.

Notwithstanding these potential benefits, considerable doubts remain about the depth of investment and overt commitment that managed care has to these public health priorities. Specific comments from one health department director highlighted this concern: "One of the biggest barriers between local health agencies and managed care plans is that plans identify community as the populations they've contracted to serve" (*State Health Watch*, 1995, p. 5).

An example of potential and challenges in addressing such barriers is how managed care plans address the public health and treatment needs of patients with tuberculosis. A report from the CDC identified components that make up any comprehensive strategy for an effective treatment, management, and community control program (Halverson and others, 1997):

• Planning and policy
• Identifying TB cases
• Managing TB cases
• Using appropriate technologies—both laboratory and diagnostic
• Application of data by a public health agency in assisting private providers to document and treat cases
• Related training and education of providers

Alliances with public health agencies around tuberculosis represent potential benefits to managed care. In some cases, state actions may work to influence the development of such relationships, including avoiding costs for more intensive treatment by reducing TB exposure and the information transfer of clinical guidelines for TB diagnosis and treatment from public health agencies to managed care plans.

California and other states have required Medicaid HMOs to establish memoranda of understanding with public health agencies on the provision of public health services to their beneficiaries. This collaboration can include physician education on TB diagnosis, service contracts for care to be delivered at public health clinics, and data sharing regarding testing and treatment. These alliances are inherently beneficial but not risk free. Problems that may arise include direct competition for vulnerable populations between these two entities, and the failure to recognize the need for coordination to control TB. However, in successful cases, public health–managed care alliances may work to influence a local network of health care providers to create a communitywide approach to screening, diagnosis, and treatment of TB and other conditions.

Physicians and Allied Health Professionals

Managed care's emphasis on comprehensive care, prevention, and coordination can strengthen the network of providers who care for inner-city residents. However, as they become the primary players in the inner city, these organizations face old, difficult problems. Issues of access to and the supply of health professionals arise, as do questions about how well community physicians will be assimilated into this framework. Ultimately these historical and current issues, which were identified as part of the inner-city ecology description in Chapter Two and are elaborated on here, point to potential areas of intervention and change that, if addressed, could significantly and positively alter the substantially flawed current nonsystem. If they are left unaddressed, managed care could worsen the situation by further excluding and neglecting needy populations in historically underserved areas.

Medicaid Physician Payments

Low Medicaid payment levels have been cited as a critical cause of inequities in access to care in the inner city. For example, low funding or lack of funding for critical health-related services such as language interpretation, child care, and transportation may make it problematic for providers to participate in managed care. Medicaid managed care needs to align the financial incentives in a way that ensures providers are adequately compensated and willing to participate.

The predominance of Medicaid combined with socioeconomic disadvantage in the inner city creates a powerful determinant, and sometimes a deterrent, for provider participation in caring for vulnerable populations. A 1997 publication presents key findings about the nonmonetary determinants of Medicaid participation among office-based primary care physicians practicing in cities (Perloff, Kletke, Fossett, and Banks, 1997). The focus of the study was to determine how factors such as Medicaid fees and community characteristics like poverty and racial segregation might affect participation. The investigators also considered if physician participation in Medicaid is affected by a community's socioeconomic characteristics and extent of racial segregation (Perloff, Kletke, Fossett, and Banks, 1997). They hypothesized that physicians practicing in more segregated cities will practice in the more prosperous areas of those cities, while those choosing lower-income areas are more likely to serve Medicaid patients and participate in Medicaid.

Using information drawn from an American Medical Association telephone survey on a sample of urban-based primary care physicians, researchers found that racial segregation, community income level, and demand from the eligible Medicaid population significantly influenced physician participation. In contrast, payment levels were not associated with Medicaid program participation. They also determined that providers who treat inner-city residents and are located in the inner city tend to be women and foreign-trained physicians. The authors concluded that strategies other than simply increasing Medicaid fees must accompany increases in Medicaid payment levels to reach the goal of equitable access, and they suggest initiatives to subsidize the creation of practices in neglected urban areas, supporting community health centers, or adding physicians and other providers to certain settings (Perloff, Kletke, Fossett, and Banks, 1997).

Provider Diversity

Diversity among professionals providing care to inner-city residents is key to reaching and serving the ethnically and culturally diverse population. A 1993 telephone survey asked 6,674 California residents to self-report access according to factors such as appointment waiting time, physician visits, travel time to regular source of care, and presence of a regular source of care (Grumbach, Vranizan, and Bindman, 1997). Researchers also calculated the ratio of physicians per 100,000 population using the American Medical Association Physician Master File data and 1994 U.S. Census figures. Findings indicated that minorities, the uninsured, and the poor tended to reside in urban areas with fewer physicians, and that these characteristics accounted for differences in access to care. The authors concluded that residing in an area with a substantial number of physicians is not necessarily related to unencumbered access if individuals are uninsured and have lower incomes. The following policy implications were drawn from this work:

- A more equitable redistribution of physicians alone will not necessarily improve access significantly among these vulnerable populations.
- Simply adding more physicians will not yield greater access.
- Selectively working to increase the number of minority physicians may be a more effective strategy.

Provider Issues with Managed Care and Implications

Assimilation of inner-city community physicians into managed care faces many challenges and obstacles. A survey of 1,710 physicians who practiced mainly in staff model HMOs indicated that the greater the percentage of their patient base who were enrolled in managed care plans, the greater the percentage of physicians who reported difficulty in referring to specialists, especially specialists of their choice (Scott-Collins, Schoen, and Sandman, 1997). According to the Survey of Physician Experiences with Managed Care, a Commonwealth Fund publication, physicians complained about the increased burden of additional administrative costs due to the need to participate in several different health plans in order to keep their patients. The report also found that black and Latino physicians were more likely to provide services to more disadvantaged patient populations.

The expansion of managed care into the inner city may introduce other more potentially serious concerns for access to care for low-income populations. Bindman and others (1998) used responses to a mail survey from 947 office-based primary care physicians in thirteen large, urban California counties to identify problems in their entry to managed care networks. Although they uncovered no pattern of discrimination based on physician's race or sex, they did find that the demographic characteristics of the patients these physicians saw were significantly related to managed care participation. In particular, greater proportions of patients who were not white or lacked insurance were associated with fewer capitated enrollees and greater likelihood of denial of managed care contracts. These findings led the authors to conclude, "Perhaps our most worrisome finding is that primary care physicians who provide a disproportionate amount of care to the uninsured and to nonwhite patients are significantly less likely to have managed care patients. Rather than rewarding these physicians for their socially responsible deeds, the health care marketplace seems to be excluding them" (Bindman and others, 1998, p. 679).

Other health care providers in the inner city also are uncertain about their role in managed care. This uncertainty injects a more immediate anxiety into the health workforce and can destabilize organizations. One study examined the nursing profession and the effects of managed care on earnings in high– and low–managed care penetration states between 1983 and 1994 (Buerhaus and Staiger, 1996). The authors found that registered nurse staffing in hospitals decreased, and the decline was more pronounced in high–managed care states than in low–managed care states. In addition, the wages of nurses had not significantly increased since 1990.

Finally, the provider community must contend with market demands and shoulder responsibility as well. Lower rates of board certification may discourage managed care organizations from contracting with physicians. Also, physicians are not being trained in how to deal with managed care and its repercussions (Bischoff and others, 1997). Researchers have highlighted the need to develop programs for this purpose and cite an effort by Jefferson Medical College, which created a one-year managed care fellowship for post-residency physicians in 1995. Among its aims, the fellowship is intended to correct misconceptions that academic medical centers and managed care organizations have about one another.

In sum, the current drive for market advantage and cost containment in the context of managed care is rearranging who delivers services in urban areas. Providers are deciding or being forced to decide whether it is feasible to participate, how they should adapt, and whether they can sustain care to vulnerable populations. In some cases, the decision is being made for them.

The Traditional Providers of Care in the Inner City and Their Integration with Managed Care

Urban safety net providers represent a potentially rich source of experience and competency in caring for inner-city residents. Some hospitals and health systems are taking advantage of their position and creating their own managed care plans. In other situations, they are becoming primary contractors for services. Still others are less certain about their fate. No matter what strategy is evolving, many of these providers face fundamental challenges and questions about their structure, governance, staffing needs, services, and ultimately their mission. Managed care plans and organizations that are not safety net based will need to decide what relationship, if any, they will have with traditional providers of care.

The following narrative reviews the potential and emerging impact of managed care on traditional providers. It highlights the organizational cultural issues, noting differences that could impede relationships. Early emerging findings from the effects of managed care highlight concerns, opportunities, and directions for traditional providers.

Contexts for Collaboration: Potential Benefits and Barriers

On the surface, the mutual benefit of collaboration between many traditional providers of care in the inner city and managed care organizations seems evident. A report prepared for the primary national organization representing managed care plans, the American Association of Health Plans, discussed in some detail the pros and cons of creating this collaboration (Orbovitch, 1996). It pointed out how managed care organizations could capitalize on the experience and geographic location of the existing service structure and traditional providers in communities, especially in caring for Medicaid enrollees. Linguistic and cultural familiarity also may fit well into their outreach, case management, and marketing objectives, and the range of social health and medical services (such as translation and nutrition supplement programs) extends beyond their typical activities. In essence, it may be more cost-effective for managed care organizations to work with community providers than to establish these important services independently.

Community-based providers, who constitute a large segment of the inner-city safety net, could benefit from collaboration in a number of ways. Managed care organizations are likely to offer additional revenue stability; increased access to specialists and other providers through the network, as well as an established process for these links; an emphasis on tracking service use and management information systems; and general technical assistance as well as educational opportunities to learn about the management of certain health conditions.

Although these potential benefits bring to the fore why such affiliations may be worthwhile, many identified barriers can significantly encumber attempts to collaborate (Orbovitch, 1996):

Organization

- Different organizational cultures, in which mission, values, and corporate language vary. For example, enabling service and support services may not match the managed care financing system or medical model.

- Questionable value of the public health model of health care delivery among some managed care organizations.
- Community-based perceptions that managed care organizations do not understand the low-income population's needs.
- Difficulty working with providers with weak administrative structures, minimal capitation financing knowledge, and less-than-optimal information and reporting systems.

Financing

- Difficulty pricing according to managed care organization methods among community providers, especially when actuarial information for underserved populations may be unavailable.
- Financial management of chronic illnesses such as HIV may be more difficult in managed care organizations, especially with rapidly changing protocols and the related changing (if not escalating) costs of drug treatment regimens.
- Questionable understanding about the key role that state government plays in determining what core medical services are covered under Medicaid.
- Inadequate methods for risk-adjusting actuarial rates to reflect a case mix of safety net providers.

Reward Systems

- Different reward systems under grant programs and managed care. Under grant programs, community-based providers measure success by counting the number of encounters. In managed care those same providers are rewarded for efficiency, reduction of visits, and emphasizing prevention and disease management. In fact, they may need to function in both worlds and to maximize both paradigms.

These benefits and barriers can be incorporated into a continuum of collaboration that represents the relationships between community-based providers and managed care organizations. Its range includes short-term cooperation on specific health efforts to full partnerships, in which organizations share a common agenda and financial risk.

Managed Care and Traditional Providers of Care: Impact and Actions

Given the potential benefits and areas of concern, how have the traditional providers of inner-city health care responded to managed care? How has managed care affected them to date? A selective review of reports to date indicates early patterns that lead in quite different, if not significantly divergent, directions of both opportunity and difficulty.

A 1997 preliminary report documented the impact of mandatory Medicaid managed care on Philadelphia's community providers, including high-volume Medicaid hospitals and federally qualified and city health centers, as well as multiservice providers such as school clinics (Hurley, Zinn, Rosko, and Kuder, 1997). The interview-based results and conclusions target areas of opportunity and concern that have relevance in other urban areas. For example, the authors found that the history of managed care has expanded choice for beneficiaries and created opportunities for participation by community providers in managed care networks, and that continuity of care improved, furthering ways to continue service to populations with special needs.

Initial fears and experiences could undermine these positive factors, however. Among the major concerns are that both public and nonprofit providers will not be able to sustain their traditional mission as managed care pressures reorient service priorities to certain enrollees and what will occur if government support for the uninsured is reduced: "As reimbursement rates are expected to be lower, the ability of organizations to subsidize services for the indigent is severely restrained" (Hurley, Zinn, Rosko, and Kuder, 1997, p. iv). This situation will be exacerbated as on-off Medicaid eligibility remains common. The fact that HMOs will not balance resource allocation adequately among medical, social, and enabling services is a vital concern for inner-city residents. Other concerns are that special needs such as mental health will be inadequately covered and that the public and school health needs of residents will be compromised if the city withdraws local support and there is a failure to reconcile the relationship of such entities with managed care organizations effectively.

Provider responses to the market changes include board education, staff layoffs, major affiliation initiatives, and recognition of a substantial lack of capital for infrastructure or management system improvement, especially among health centers. Some providers have noted the poor level of education about managed care among Medicaid enrollees, resulting in inappropriate use of providers. One hospital noted that its layoffs "were directly the result of growing demand for care from uninsured persons" (Hurley, Zinn, Rosko, and Kuder, 1997, p. 19).

Medicaid Managed Care in Texas
Texas Bureau of Medicaid Interview

Texas initiated a Medicaid managed care pilot project in 1993 in the Austin and Galveston regions. In September 1996, the program was formalized and expanded to the cities and surrounding counties of San Antonio, Fort Worth, and Lubbock. The most recent phase of the expansion, in late 1997, was to the city of Houston and the surrounding area.

A goal of Texas's Medicaid managed care program is to contract competitively in these specific geographical areas for the TANF (Temporary Assistance to Needy Families) population for physical and behavioral health. In the Houston area, the SSI population (Supplemental Security Income, for example, the disabled qualifying for Medicaid) is also covered by three of the participating

HMOs. In areas where Medicaid managed care is mandated, enrollees choose between an HMO option and a primary care case management (PCCM) option. In selecting the HMOs to participate in the program, the state uses rigorous procurement methods to ensure a competitive selection process.

In San Antonio, the majority (63 percent) of the Medicaid population was enrolled in the primary care case management model in 1997. The remainder of the Aid for Dependent Children (AFDC) population was enrolled in three managed care plans. The most successful of the plans in San Antonio is sponsored by the San Antonio Hospital District. In 1995, it obtained this contract by successfully participating in the bidding process.

The Harris County Hospital District was initially unsuccessful in competing for a Medicaid managed care contract. It is the largest safety net provider in Houston and includes two hospitals and a network of ambulatory care sites. It is also the largest provider of indigent care in Houston and a major Medicaid provider; in 1995 its Medicaid net patient revenues exceeded $170 million. However, when the managed care procurement took place in mid-1997, the Harris County Hospital District bid did not secure a contract. Fundamental questions were raised regarding the future of the safety net in Houston and whether the county hospital district should receive special consideration during the contract process. Analysis by the district indicated that the hospital would lose tens of millions of dollars if it did not get a contract, a situation that would result in increases to county taxes. Coincidental with the bidding process, the Texas legislature was in session and passed legislation mandating that hospital districts could be managed care plans if they could successfully meet the managed care contract terms.

Following passage of the legislation, the Harris County Hospital District obtained a Medicaid managed care contract. After the contract was awarded, the hospital district received both telephone and on-site technical assistance from the Department of Health to bring the county program into conformity with state requirements.

Questions still remain as to whether the hospital will be successful as a managed care plan.

Hospitals

Given the focus and financial concentration on inpatient care, hospitals may face the greatest challenges of all providers in adapting to managed care. Such difficulties were profiled in recent California reports. In one study, investigators found that between 1983 and 1993, hospital expenditure increases were 44 percent lower in areas with high HMO penetration compared with those in low-penetration markets and that outpatient utilization often was substituted for inpatient care (Robinson, 1996). The report concluded, "Managed care is shifting the acute care hospital from the center toward the periphery of the health care system" (p. 1060). A 1997 study documented the change in the number of public hospitals. In 1964 California had sixty-eight public hospitals, located in forty-nine of the state's fifty-eight counties; by 1997 that number had declined over 50 percent to twenty-four hospitals in seventeen counties (Pope, 1995). Some projections are that the state's public hospitals are "doomed" due to overbedding, Medi-Cal competition, and managed care. The alternative may very well be a private system with county support.

One dramatic example of the impact of marketing and care to the poor is seen in El Paso, Texas. The *New York Times* reported ("Hospitals Serving the Poor . . . ," 1997) that the increasing competition for Medicaid patients there is leaving the local public hospital with greater numbers of illegal immigrants, patients suffering from drug abuse, and other vulnerable populations, while patients with insurance are enticed to private hospitals or health centers. This public provider, Thomason Hospital, the only not-for-profit provider in the community, experienced an increase in its uninsured patient population as a percentage of its total population from 40 percent to 47 percent in a few years, while the Medicaid proportion declined from 39 percent to 34 percent. One of the hardest-hit areas is obstetrics, where Thomason Hospital has seen a 16 percent Medicaid decrease since 1993.

Causes for concern are arising in other urban areas as well. An update on the impact of the Tenncare program in Tennessee cited the continued uncertainty and potential adverse impact on the major urban safety net hospital in Memphis, the Regional Center of Memphis (MED) (Gold, Frazer, and Schoen, 1995). In only a few years, the MED experienced a drop in deliveries from 8,000 to 3,500 per year, the number of medical residents in training decreased from 140 to 110, and the institution reduced its beds by 200. A 1997 study (Center for Workforce Studies, 1997) on the marketplace and health system in New York City documented that between 1995 and 2000, as many as 32 percent of the city's beds may close and over thirty-six thousand jobs (20 percent of all full-time equivalents) may be lost (subject to the pace that managed care is implemented in the state).

Concern over the impact of managed care has led to speculation that emergency departments (EDs) may close due to the financial burden placed on hospitals. ED financial instability is caused in part by retroactive refusals to pay for care by managed care organizations. Compounding this situation is the likelihood that fewer Medicaid visits will lead to a decreased ability to cost-shift, leaving hospitals without the means to cover their losses for treating the uninsured. Hospitals' responses include alleviating the financial pressures and demand from uninsured patients to more effective triage of patients.

Responses from Urban Safety Net Hospitals

Certain public sector providers have taken advantage of the impetus generated by managed care to enact constructive and potentially significant health care system changes for their infrastructures, general populations, and targeted vulnerable populations such as the uninsured. For example, the county-owned program in and around Indianapolis, Wishard Advantage, has targeted individuals with incomes up to 200 percent of poverty to participate as commercial and Medicaid managed care enrollees (Jaklevic, 1997). This population has access to all in-system services and providers. Challenges to the public system are to entice these patients into Wishard and not to create disincentives for enrolling in other health insurance programs, especially since the corporation that oversees Wishard Advantage estimates its indigent care costs are $65 million annually. At least five other public settings—Contra Costa County in California, Cooper Green Hospital in Birmingham, Harborview Medical Center in Seattle, and Metropolitan Health Plan in Minneapolis and in Tampa, Florida—have developed similar programs for the indigent.

In 1997 a system of outpatient clinics and the University of Texas Health Science Center in San Antonio initiated a managed care program, called CareLink, for the uninsured in its surrounding urban area (*State Health Watch*, 1997). This program provides enrollees with access to primary care and other services within this inpatient and ambulatory care system. Key objectives include reducing waiting time, improving satisfaction, gaining cost control, and establishing seamlessness in care between Medicaid and the uninsured.

To serve an acutely ill population better, New York City's Harlem Hospital created a managed care program for Medicaid patients in 1992 (Goldman 1993). The program is based on twelve principles:

1. Each enrollee is linked to a primary care physician (PCP).
2. Each PCP accepts responsibility for coordinating all enrollee health care services.
3. Each PCP must preapprove all enrollee services.
4. The PCP must participate in twenty-four-hour telephone coverage.
5. The PCPs are organized into teams, each of which will manage a panel of twenty-five hundred patients.

6. PCP teams contain a physician, a nurse practitioner, and/ or a physician assistant.

7. The physician team member is ultimately responsible for all patients assigned to the team's panel.

8. To ensure availability and continuity of care, each physician must conduct at least five outpatient sessions per week, including at least one evening or weekend session.

9. The team's schedule must allow for both scheduled and walk-in patients.

10. Patients who present in the ED and are not urgent and patients who self-refer for specialty services will be directed to their teams.

11. All physicians are required to participate in the inpatient care of their patients.

12. Each physician must participate in all quality improvement, peer review, and all other administrative functions.

University Hospital of Medicine and Dentistry in Newark, New Jersey, established a private group teaching practice for women's health services (Loughlin, Bronner, and Mascare, 1997). Its practice goal was to attract more Medicaid obstetrical patients and to serve as a model for other ambulatory care services that the hospital offered. In 1995 the obstetrics department established a continuity-of-care demonstration project to enhance the educational experience of residents and the quality of patient care. Patient education on health promotion and disease-specific care information also became a key component in patient treatment.

Finally, some hospitals have concentrated their efforts and finances on transforming into integrated delivery systems (IDS) (Bennett and Young, 1997). One author points out that public hospitals in particular face many barriers when establishing IDSs. They must adapt to some treatments being provided outside the hospital and consequently may be relegated to providing the second tier of care in the delivery system. They also need to recruit a sufficient number of physicians who understand managed care and will serve as gatekeepers. Other challenges stem from the fact that organizational control of public hospitals, civil service requirements, lack of capital, and strong labor unions traditionally have not been consistent with IDS management style, which requires a high degree of flexibility.

Community Health Programs

One response to the inner cities' health care access problems in the 1960s was the establishment by the federal government of community health centers that targeted poor and underserved populations. Forty percent of the approximately six hundred centers, caring for about 6 million people, are in impoverished inner-city areas (Physician Payment Review Commission, 1994). Their objectives are provision of primary care, education, screening, and care for high-prevalence conditions such as infant mortality, hypertension, and cardiovascular conditions, and redirecting individuals away from more expensive sites, such as EDs.

Community health centers cared for almost 9 million patients in 1994, an increase of over 25 percent since 1990 according to the National Association of Community Health Centers (1995). Approximately 44 percent of their service population is under nineteen years old; 30 percent are women in childbearing years. An estimated 60 percent live in poor areas, and a similar percentage have income below the federal poverty level (U.S. General Accounting Office, 1995).

Examples of community health centers include Roxbury Comprehensive Community Health Center, Roxbury, Massachusetts. The center, founded in 1969, is located a few miles from downtown Boston in a densely populated neighborhood. Poverty and unemployment have plagued the neighborhood for decades. The clinic now has two community sites, ten departments, and a full complement of primary care physicians, midlevel practitioners, and other clinical personnel. The majority of the patient population is children and adolescents. The center serves more than ten thousand people with more than fifty thousand medical encounters annually. Another center is Northeast Medical Services in San Francisco, formed over twenty years ago by a group of concerned citizens. The health center was developed to respond to critical health care problems associated with inner-city poverty and unemployment. Today the center serves a primarily Asian population, including many new immigrants (Gage and others, 1996).

Despite these promising examples, the future of urban community health centers under managed care is unclear. Their focus on ambulatory and primary care, their location in the community, and their frequently long-standing relationship with the community make them especially attractive as participants in managed care networks (Pope, 1995). According to a U.S. General Accounting Office report (1995), 500,000 community health center patients were already enrolled in primarily Medicaid managed care programs in 1993, a 55 percent increase in only two years.

At the same time, changes in the health care system have left community health centers vulnerable during the transition to managed care, since they have limited resources to compete for patients on a level with private HMOs (Schauffler and Wolin, 1996). Although most community health centers are managing to remain open, they are feeling financially threatened by the prepaid capitated payment rates dictated by Medicaid managed care (GAO, 1995). As of the early to mid-1990s, fewer than one-fourth of the centers had entered contract relationships with managed care providers or been designated as such. In reviewing the impact of managed care on ten community health centers, the GAO found that all had increased their patient caseload and generally improved their financial bottom line (three reported managed care–related losses). Seven had been able to increase the resources for uncompensated care. Nonetheless, the report concluded that because of low capitation rates, assumption of financial risk exceeding their capacity, and insufficient information, experience, and knowledge about managed care, these programs may be in jeopardy. In fact, the

GAO reported that one center had to curtail services because it faced insolvency.

Assessments on the future conclude that these centers will need technical assistance and new infrastructure to compete in a managed care environment (Schauffler and Wolin, 1996). In particular, they will need to find additional funding sources for their continued viability. None of the clinics that the U.S. General Accounting Office reviewed had sufficient cash on hand to meet the Bureau of Primary Health Care's suggested financial viability benchmark. The clinics have maintained their service levels but have encountered great financial difficulties, especially since the introduction of managed care.

The Wellness Plan, Detroit, Michigan
An Interview with Isadore King, executive director

The Wellness Plan (TWP) is a successor plan to the federally sponsored model neighborhood–model cities program from the late 1960s. In 1972 it became a licensed HMO. Current enrollment is approximately 150,000, 89 percent of whom have Medicaid, 10 percent commercial coverage, and 1 percent Medicare. TWP is a mixed-model HMO that owns and operates four health care centers that are not federally funded. A staff of seventy full-time equivalent (FTE) physicians offer a range of ambulatory services, as well as pharmacy, laboratory, outpatient surgery, primary care, and radiology. They also have contracts with local medical groups, independent provider associations of private physicians, and contracts with individual physicians. Inpatient care is provided through contracts with over forty hospitals.

TWP faces a number of future challenges. One of them is having Medicaid as the primary purchaser because 3 percent of Medicaid enrollees lose coverage each month. The entire population turns over at least every three years. In addition, TWP finds that it is impossible to separate social issues from the health issues that affect inner-city residents. Significant social issues include lack of transportation, malnutrition, low income, substandard housing, substance abuse, low literacy, and other socioeconomic factors that impede many enrollees from taking responsibility for their health status. To address this issue, TWP finds a continuing need for patient education, consumer advocacy, and community service.

To be effective in providing care to a Medicaid population, TWP believes that it has to maintain a public health service system perspective, which includes the development of collaborative community programs, adopting a school, and, through that relationship, supporting a teen health center. In addition, there is a need to form collaborative relationships between the public and private sectors to eliminate possible service duplication in the areas of care to children, immunizations, and prenatal care. For example, the local public health departments provide services also provided by TWP.

TWP is facing reduced margins due to lower Medicaid and commercial premiums and increasing medical and administrative expenses. A main method for plans such as TWP to survive financially is to serve larger patient volumes and achieve a different purchaser mix. To remain successful, over the next five years, TWP anticipates serving a larger commercial and Medicare market, while maintaining its commitment to the Medicaid population.

Internal Adaptation

One fear emerging from this sector of the safety net is that managed care organizations not affiliated with community health centers may move into urban markets and usurp the paying patient base, leaving facilities with little capital for the competitive market and higher-risk patients or a greater proportion of uninsured patients. Moreover, waivers and other modifications to Medicaid in many states have reduced government support and created greater uncertainty about the ability of community health centers to sustain both their mission and financial viability.

Another fear is that their inability to maintain financial independence will lead to a subsuming under academic medical institutions or large hospitals. While not inherently adverse in the effect on patients, some of these organizations may be eager to capture "trophy centers" that give the appearance of creating a community link but where the center only serves as a patient "feeder" for the hospital.

To counteract these concerns, community health centers are undertaking a variety of actions, sometimes in combination. These include integrated service networks that involve centers and other service entities, HMO subcontracts, and developing state relationships that promote their role as case managers. In certain cases (for example, Oregon), states have taken at least some action to require managed care entities to include community health centers and other traditional health care providers (such as public health clinics) in the delivery of certain services such as immunizations and communicable disease treatment. These and other initiatives take on greater importance as cost-based reimbursement is essentially being phased out.

A 1998 *Washington Post* article highlighted the cost of increased competition for community health centers in Newark. The report, headlined "Health Care Safety Net Is Fraying," notes how community health centers experienced an 11 percent decrease in Medicaid patients between 1995 and 1996 and a 14 percent increase in the uninsured ("Clinics Losing Ground . . . ," 1998). Reasons for this change include misreading the market by believing that their experience would identify them as almost irresistible partners to managed care organizations new to the urban and Medicaid markets, signing with only a few HMOs, and needing higher negotiated rates based on the desire to include enabling services such as transportation.

Those most familiar with the situation of community health centers indicate that their greatest challenge is to understand and adapt to the business of health care. This includes learning to balance the social mission with increasing budget limitations. For example, many managed care organizations currently court community health centers as partners for managed care. However, many community providers believe that the managed care organizations are interested solely in the patient population for referrals, and have little actual interest in learning more about the needs of inner-city populations. In these instances, managed care organizations' true objectives may simply be either to capture the health center patient base or remain in the partnership for a few months before moving on to other partners. Community health centers need to implement practice guidelines and cost-cutting measures to become viable partners. According to some, many community health centers are moving too slowly to adapt effectively to needed changes. Others in a number of locations are learning quickly and may do quite well.

Nonetheless, it is likely that a sizable proportion of community health centers will face consolidation in the future. Although the needs of their communities are not being met, the almost one thousand organizations with three thousand delivery sites will not likely sustain the financial and competitive pressures. At the same time, consolidation is a double-edged sword: it creates better-run and more viable community health centers, but it also reduces the total number of clinics and therefore threatens to reduce access.

Conclusion

In a turbulent environment where competition may not easily beget collaboration, the alliance of managed care with traditional providers of care in urban areas, especially those whose mission has focused on care for vulnerable populations, is far from easy. Still, success for both sectors may depend on their ability to forge these relationships, with the health of these communities at ultimate stake. Each sector brings strengths to urban health care; nevertheless, many critical questions require response.

Managed care plans must determine the fit of public health within their business objectives and mission. Collaboration with public health to address communitywide and systemwide concerns such as communicable diseases is a critical relationship for improving the health of inner-city residents. It may also provide an opportunity to coordinate managed care operations and systems expertise with the experience of those with broad knowledge in treating inner-city conditions. For inner-city providers, managed care offers significant incentives for collaboration. The advantages for providers include revenue stability, an established network, more emphasis on tracking and information systems, and technical assistance. Traditional community providers offer managed care organizations location, familiarity with populations, service networks, and the Medicaid patient base. At this time, the shape of this relationship is evolving and far from clear in many urban communities.

A growing concern around the impact of managed care in the inner city is the availability of physicians. This is not a simple variation on the current supply and demand and excess physician capacity discussions. Rather, this is a fundamental distribution problem that can be dangerously misleading if adequacy is based primarily on physician numbers in a city and not where those physicians are willing to practice.

Many factors influence adequacy in numbers and the access to medical professionals for urban residents located in underserved areas. Low Medicaid physician payment levels and socioeconomic characteristics of the community can interact as powerful codeterrents in caring for inner-city low-income residents. Many physicians who care for vulnerable populations in the inner city may find it increasingly difficult, if not impossible, to maintain their mission within the competitive managed care model. With managed care financing affecting health care delivery, many physicians are both untrained about how to work within its financial requirements and unsure about their ability to sustain an inner-city practice. Compounding the difficulties of physicians who care for the uninsured and minority patients in the inner city is evidence that they may face a greater likelihood of not being accepted as participating providers by managed care plans.

Minority physicians tend to practice more often in the more financially depressed communities and to see greater numbers of minority patients. Thus, building the capacity and numbers of this provider group may be a critical component to any efforts by managed care plans to ensure adequate access in these urban areas. However, there is no clear indication that the numbers of minority physicians graduating from medical school will approach the demand for services in these areas. Thus, policies that create additional incentives for minority practices in these areas and recruitment of minorities into medical school could work to alleviate these problems, but lack of such directed efforts as well as anti-affirmative action efforts could sabotage the little progress that has been made.

While community providers—both organization and physicians—and managed care could benefit from collaboration, significant barriers encumber such efforts. Most relevant are differences in organizational cultures, unfamiliarity with the managed care financing model among traditional providers, mutual perceptions about value, the need for substantial administrative system development by many community providers, various financing issues related to pricing services, roles of government as perceived by managed care, and historically different reward systems. Of particular concern to the hospitals is the profound shift in service delivery from an acute, inpatient care focus to primary and clinic-based care. The ability for the majority to make a financially and organizationally successful transition is far from certain.

Finally, the fate of safety net providers regarding their managed care role is a very mixed evolution. Some have achieved success in their own right by developing managed care plans, others are primarily contracting with these organizations, and some are still evaluating strategic alternatives. These different efforts portend varied outcomes, with scenarios ranging from successful integration into managed care delivery systems to closure or absorption into larger provider organizations. The looming questions are how each outcome will affect the quality of and access to services in urban communities and, ultimately, who will participate in deciding the fate of these providers.

Chapter Four

Integrating Urban Teaching Hospitals into Managed Care

The previous chapter described the effect of managed care on traditional providers of care. This chapter reviews the impact of managed care on teaching hospitals and their affiliated medical schools and describes how these institutions are responding. This relationship is important to document because many of these organizations and their affiliates are located in the inner city and provide significant volumes of services to local residents. They play important national and local roles related to conducting basic and clinical medical research, as well as for training future physicians. Managed care's evolution in the inner city has potentially major consequences for the scope, direction, and volume related to all three roles that are core to the mission of urban teaching hospitals. In essence, these institutions must reconsider each of these core activities and, essentially, the role of the academic medical center itself.

This chapter considers the academic medical center's capacity to preserve its mission in the context of managed care. In addition to our review and synthesis of information from literature and interviews, we incorporated results from a national survey. To study the relationship between managed care and teaching hospitals, we surveyed 330 primarily urban-based teaching hospitals that are members of the National Association of Public Hospitals and Health Systems or the Association of American Medical Colleges' Council of Teaching Hospitals. (Appendix A contains a description of the survey methods and the questionnaire used.) The Teaching Hospital Survey on Managed Care in Urban Areas, conducted in 1997, examined the impact of managed care on teaching hospitals

from five perspectives: revenue effects, affiliations and service contracting, extent of managed care involvement, workforce and physician specialty areas, and utilization.

Two assumptions formed the survey content areas and objectives. First, we believed that the desired balance between managed
care and teaching hospitals should be one of increased efficiency
and improved patient satisfaction while maintaining the mission of
the institutions. Second, we concluded that to achieve this balance,
organizations must be willing to change, have available the capital
needed to make necessary changes, and must resolve the challenges
of financing for care to the uninsured.

The results report responses from 117 hospitals for 1996. Because this group represents only 40 percent of the membership universe, we view these results with some caution. Nonetheless, the
responses were regionally representative of that universe, with similar numbers of public and private hospitals reporting. Our conclusion is that these findings, brought together with other information,
offer a profile of a key inner-city service sector struggling to adjust
to a rapidly shifting health care environment.

Old Questions, New Issues for Urban Teaching
Hospitals and Their Medical Schools

The survey and literature show that managed care is reducing financial support to urban teaching hospitals and their affiliated medical
schools. This financial stress can either stimulate change or weaken
an organization. Recent findings by the Task Force on Academic
Health Centers highlight the dependence of academic health centers (AHCs) on clinical revenues to support their social mission
and how these missions raise costs. Funding of AHCs to serve vulnerable populations is an important factor that influences their ability to compete in private markets. These hospitals are especially
affected by changes occurring in Medicare and Medicaid reimbursement policies. In 1996 61 percent of total net revenues at
public hospitals came from Medicare and Medicaid (National Asso-

ciation of Public Hospitals, 1998). In 1994 private academic health centers derived 48 percent of their revenues from Medicare and Medicaid (Reuter, 1997). If expansion of Medicare and Medicaid managed care results in reductions to revenues at teaching hospitals, change will need to occur.

These two public insurance programs are rapidly phasing in managed care reimbursement policies. Medicare beneficiaries currently have a choice of whether they want to enroll in managed care, and the majority are still selecting fee-for-service. However, the number of elderly enrolled in HMOs is expected to grow during the next five years, assuming that these organizations continue to see this population as profitable—a far from certain assumption. In 1996 11 percent of Medicare beneficiaries, or 4.3 million, were enrolled in risk plans. This figure is expected to double by 2002. The Medicaid program has increased the use of managed care, and in many states recipients are required to select a managed care option. From 1990 to 1996 the number of Medicaid recipients enrolled in managed care plans grew from 2.3 million to 13.3 million, accounting for 40 percent of all Medicaid recipients.

For teaching hospitals to maintain their revenue base, they must receive sufficient revenues from Medicare and Medicaid so that they can continue their educational programs, research, and care to the underinsured and uninsured. To date, however, substantial Medicare and Medicaid managed care penetration rates are not reflected in teaching hospitals' revenues. As of 1997, the impact of managed care on teaching hospitals as reported in the survey only began to emerge, with half of the responding hospitals receiving less than 20 percent of their revenues from managed care. As seen in Table 4.1, responding public hospitals documented even less of a relationship with managed care, with 41 percent deriving less than 5 percent of their patient revenues from managed care and only 19 percent of public hospitals deriving 6 to 10 percent of their revenues from such affiliations.

For this period, 55 percent of respondents reported that the number of beneficiaries with commercial insurance had decreased,

**Table 4.1. Percentage of Patient Revenues Derived
from Managed Care Contracts, by Ownership**

Patient Revenues	Public Hospitals		Private Hospitals	
	Year 1996	Year 2000	Year 1996	Year 2000
<5%	41% (24)	2% (1)	0%	0%
6–10%	19% (11)	9% (5)	5% (3)	0%
11–20%	17% (10)	20% (11)	21% (12)	4% (2)
21–30%	14% (8)	13% (7)	41% (23)	4% (2)
31–50%	7% (4)	36% (20)	23% (13)	65% (35)
51–75%	2% (1)	21% (12)	9% (5)	22% (12)
75–100%	0%	0%	0%	6% (3)

Source: Teaching Hospital Survey on Managed Care in Urban Areas.
Note: $p < 0.01$, $X^2 = 43$, DF = 5 for 1996.

and 42 percent reported that the number of Medicaid patients had decreased. The survey documents that proportionately more responding public hospitals associate considerable portions of their patient charges with self-pay, charity, or uninsured: 57 percent of responding public hospitals related 21 to 75 percent of their charges with these patients. The majority of responding private hospitals, 79 percent, associate up to 10 percent of their charges from self-pay, charity, or uninsured. The report of the Commonwealth Fund on academic health centers (Reuter, 1997b) reinforces this result, finding that teaching hospitals are assuming an increasing burden of uncompensated care. They reported that from 1989 to 1994, uncompensated care rose by 26 percent in AHC hospitals, from 9.3 percent to 11.7 percent of gross patient revenues. However, growth in uncompensated care has not been the same in all hospital markets, and there may be some correlation with managed care penetration. In areas with high HMO enrollment, the share of uncompensated care borne by AHCs grew from 30 percent to 35 percent. between 1985 and 1993; for AHCs in areas with low HMO enrollment, the percentage remained constant (Reuter, 1997b). Public hospitals receive subsidies from state and local sources, which partially offset their uncompensated care burden; however, the uncompensated care burden at public hospitals is still higher than at other comparable hospitals (Reuter, 1997b). Furthermore, public subsidies are shrinking. The survey information documented that from 1994 to 1996 a slight majority of urban-based hospitals (51 percent) experienced increases in the percentage of uninsured patients; nevertheless, 59 percent reported a decrease in available funds for financing uninsured patients. These changes are described in Table 4.2.

AHCs are also concerned that they may be losing more profitable, lower-risk patients to other providers through their managed care plans, leaving the more costly patients for teaching hospitals (Reuter, 1997b). A recent study also suggests that safety net hospitals lost low-risk Medicaid maternity patients, while high-risk maternity patients remained concentrated in safety net hospitals (Gaskins, Hadley, and Freeman, 1998).

Table 4.2. Change in Percentage of Uninsured Using AHCs

	Increased	No Change	Decreased	Total Responding Hospitals
Uninsured patients who use hospital	50.9% (57)	44.6% (50)	4.5% (5)	112
Available funds for financing uninsured patients	9.8% (11)	31.0% (35)	59.3% (67)	113

Source: Teaching Hospital Survey on Managed Care in Urban Areas.

In the face of possible erosion of market share, teaching hospitals face special challenges in maintaining their core activities because such care is expensive and treatment protocols are not always con-sistent with the goals and processes of managed care (Pardes, 1997). At a time when managed care penetration is increasing, the uncom-pensated care burden that teaching hospitals shoulder may also be increasing. Many teaching hospitals have to reconsider core activ-ities and, essentially, the role of the institution in the community to maximize the interdependent relationships between managed care and patient care, education, and research. As a result, tensions within academic medical centers are occurring between the medical school and the affiliated hospital (Burrow, 1993). Pressure can occur at several levels: the need to provide education and research versus operating as a low-cost provider, the need to provide specialty training versus the market pressure for primary care, and the need to fill beds versus providing the shortest stays possible.

Urban Teaching Hospitals and Managed Care: Results from a National Survey

Many teaching hospitals are responding to their changing circum-stances by making changes in their delivery systems. Our survey doc-umented that to compete in a managed care environment, many academic health centers forecast improvements in infrastructure, primary care capacity, and community facility developments, but do foresee reductions in residency programs, nonphysician staff, and beds. Researchers (Caper and Fargason, 1996) have identified sev-eral management approaches to academic health centers as they seek to adapt their traditional research, education, and clinical care activities to the managed care environment. The most traditional ones—high research priority in biomedical and clinical fields, broad medical education activities, and comprehensive and quality clini-cal care—are likely to give way to one of two approaches. The first approach is a more narrowed "boutique" clinical services approach. Under this initiative, organizations opt for more focused biomedical research and tertiary care training, with patient care provided through community-based collaboration. The second alternative is a model stressing competitive primary and secondary clinical and health services, and primary care medical education.

AHCs are exploring linkages beyond the campus that are likely to be central to both of these approaches. The need for urban-based academic health centers to find more community-based primary care sites for training has combined with the need for community health centers to employ more primary care physicians to create new alliances (Reddington, Lippincott, Lindsay, and Wones, 1995). For example, the Lincoln Heights Health Center in Cincinnati, whose clients are predominantly low-income black residents, joined with the University of Cincinnati Medical Center to supplement primary care services and to improve quality, while the medical center was able to establish an out-of-hospital training site. In some circumstances, the collaboration extends directly into the community. The Johns Hopkins Medical Institutions formed partnerships with members of the East Baltimore community, including Clergy United for Renewal of East Baltimore, the Baltimore City Health Department, the school system, and Health Care for the Homeless (Levine and others, 1994). Such arrangements could be particularly beneficial for teaching hospitals in reaching underserved inner-city populations and increasing market share. In other cases, these organizations are collaborating with other health institutions, while selling off some of their buildings and resources in the face of increasing cost-cutting pressure from managed care and from lower payment rates (Managed Care Monitor, 1997).

Special Challenges for Public Teaching Hospitals

Public teaching hospitals will need to make certain strategic and organizational changes if they are to capture managed care revenues. A 1996 article (Zall, 1996) on public teaching hospitals identified several factors likely to influence greatly the future of these institutions: the age of many physical plants, the consequences of high ambulatory volume (such as long waiting times for service), federal regulatory constraints, aggressive market forces, experimentation with the Medicaid program, emphasis on managed care, and pressure to reduce beds. The public hospital systems are poorly prepared to compete effectively due to weak financial position, physical plant problems, and cumbersome governance structures. The recommendations that stem from this review focus on refashioning community-based systems and collaborating with other safety net providers. Pressure to reduce beds and to relieve the pressure on outpatient departments will require reducing inpatient staff as well, including physicians in training and the physicians training them. The reorientation toward community-based services, with the attendant shift to primary care, will call for public teaching hospitals either to affiliate with other providers of such care or to promote the development of community clinics within their own system. Their choices will be to work within their AHCs to adapt to this shift, or to bypass them by employing primary care and community-oriented physicians directly (Zall, 1996).

Survey responses further documented how hospitals were responding to managed care through organizational actions, but also confirmed the difficult challenges facing public institutions in particular. Results of selective bivariate analyses point out significant differences between urban-based public and private hospitals in the kinds of strategies that AHCs are using or planning to undertake in the light of increased competition. These findings generally suggest that urban-based public hospitals are lagging behind their private counterparts in adjusting to managed care. For example, the survey results indicated that more private hospitals own medical practices in the community and contract with managed care plans.

Organizational Redirection

The majority of reporting urban-based hospitals anticipate several important changes and redirections occurring by the year 2000 to increase efficiency and respond to lower physician demand. These actions forecast a teaching institution that is smaller than its historical proportions: reducing the numbers of beds, downsizing nonphysician staff, and shrinking residency programs (Table 4.3). To create a more advantageous position for managed care, the majority of responding urban-based hospitals anticipate that they will develop community facilities, improve systems and infrastructure, increase primary care capacity, market specialty networks, and start new capital projects (Table 4.3 gives specific percentages).

Hospitals that are implementing managed care often require capital and information systems. To raise capital and make quick decisions regarding information systems requires an institution to be organizationally nimble. The survey found an increasing awareness among many urban teaching hospitals that such needs will require fundamental restructuring. Twenty-seven percent of the responding hospitals have changed their governance during the past five years. However, these changes have not been sufficient; 56 percent still indicate a need for a major structural change in the

Table 4.3. Organizational Changes Anticipated in the Next Two Years

	Will Happen/ Likely to Happen	Unlikely to Happen/ Will Not Happen
Close beds	60.5% (69)	32.4% (37)
Develop community-based satellite facilities	86.8% (98)	10.7% (12)
Downsize medical staff	34.2% (39)	56.2% (64)
Downsize nonphysician staff	71.1% (79)	21.6% (24)
Downsize residency programs	57.1% (64)	32.2% (36)
Improve systems and infrastructure	100.0% (104)	(0)
Increase primary care capacity	93.8% (107)	5.3% (6)
Market specialty networks	89.2% (99)	4.5% (5)
New capital projects	86.8% (99)	8.8% (10)

Source: Teaching Hospital Survey on Managed Care in Urban Areas.

next two years. The hospitals that are most likely to undergo major structural changes are in markets where managed care is emerging and has not fully penetrated the market.

Delivery System Changes

Faced with increased competition for patients and the pressures to reduce costs, some AHCs are responding by instituting major changes to their services and service affiliations and by controlling their growth in expenditures. AHCs are striving to transform themselves into integrated delivery systems with the ability to provide a full range of services and to bid for managed care business. In particular, they are striving to build community-based primary care networks and to ally with physicians. Each of the following sections identifies contracting and service areas that are relevant to business imperatives and to populations served.

Specific Service Contracts. The survey found that the majority of responding urban-based hospitals (range, 59 percent to 93 percent) own the components of an integrated health delivery system. Responding hospitals have a variety of arrangements for providing ambulatory care, a core component of that system:

- Eighty-six percent reported owning or contracting with clinics.
- Eighty-two percent owned or contacted with physicians who practice in the community.
- Ninety-eight percent owned or contracted for primary care in the hospital.
- Eighty-eight percent owned or contracted for public health services. Questions were not asked about specific service volumes.
- The majority of urban-based hospitals (85 percent) owned or contracted with HMOs.

Community Physician Practices. Location of physician practices in the community is one of the key characteristics of ready adaptation to managed care. To determine how the traditional safety net providers, particularly public hospitals, are adjusting to managed care; they were compared to private hospitals. Summary responses indicate that:

- Proportionately more private hospitals, 84 percent (42 of 50), own physician practices in the community, compared with 51 percent (20 of 39) of public hospitals.
- Proportionately more public hospitals contract for physician service, 28 percent (11 of 39), compared with 8 percent (4 of 50) of private hospitals.
- Proportionately more public hospitals plan to create or buy these practices, 21 percent (8 of 39), than private hospitals, 8 percent (4 of 50). These distributions are statistically significant.

Health-Related Assistance Services. Beyond having integrated clinical services, an integrated delivery system that serves inner-city patients needs to offer critical health-related assistance and support services. The surveyed hospitals offer or contract for a variety of assistance services that supplement clinical services:

- Most responding hospitals provide counseling for domestic violence (77 percent).
- Most responding hospitals provide cultural sensitivity training for staff (87 percent) and interpreter or translator services (68 percent).
- The majority of hospitals provide public health services (64 percent) and violence-prevention programs (62 percent).
- The majority of responding urban-based hospitals directly provide or contract for transportation (74 percent) and WIC services (66 percent).

- The majority of responding hospitals do not provide assistance in obtaining housing for patients (52 percent), child care (76 percent), or homeless assistance outreach (55 percent).

Case Management. Case management, defined as an organized program that coordinates individual patient care throughout the entire spectrum of services with the goal of providing quality care in the most effective manner, is critical for managing utilization of health services. Hillman, Goldfarb, Eisenberg, and Kelley (1991), who studied urban academic medical centers' use of case management, document this need for case management. They found special challenges in changing from a fee-for-service to a managed care reimbursement structure for Medicaid. To address these challenges, a Philadelphia AHC assigned beneficiaries to faculty-level physicians who acted as gatekeepers. These physicians provided broader continuity of care and case management to patients even though the majority of physicians' time was focused on inpatient care priorities and supervision.

The survey documents that more than half the hospitals offered some type of case management services. Overall the vast majority of hospitals directly provide case management for the following services:

- Complex medical cases (74 percent)
- Patients with HIV/AIDS (73 percent)
- Nonurgent use of the emergency room (54 percent)
- Patients with mental illness (59 percent)
- Pediatric patients with chronic illness (56 percent)

In conclusion, the survey-based information and the literature portray urban teaching hospitals as undertaking a range of organization and service adaptation while still adhering to their broader mission. Evidence on restructuring indicates that many institutions see some fundamental change as essential in the process. At the same time, public hospitals may not be keeping pace with certain important changes. However, the ultimate impact of these different rates of change remains to be seen.

Managed Care and Teaching Hospital Medical Education and Research Activities

The tension between the traditional urban teaching hospital orientation and managed care's objectives threatens to create a divisive gap that could affect the research and education missions of these providers. In 1993 total graduate medical education expenditures for AHCs in high-enrollment managed care areas were 22 percent lower than in low-enrollment areas, and the gap is widening. Between 1990 and 1993 the annual rate of growth for graduate medical education spending at AHC hospitals in markets with high HMO enrollment was 7 percent, compared with 11 percent for AHCs in markets with low HMO enrollment (Reuter, 1997b). Many reasons could account for this effect, including higher costs associated with teaching hospitals generally. Published reports address the differences in objectives directly (Gold, 1998). Site visits to AHCs in three major cities during 1994 found that managed care plans were not only rarely reimbursing higher costs related to these institutions but that they also were questioning the mission of AHCs (Gold, 1998). According to the report, "Managed care plans perceive that academic medical centers are training the wrong physicians, in the wrong specialties, and in the wrong settings" (p. 280).

Academic health care centers frequently have been very slow in using managed care sites to familiarize students with managed care demands and incentives. One study of hospitals with teaching programs considered the training that residents receive in a managed care setting (Veloski and others, 1996). The authors found that managed care organization representatives did describe what they believed were the physician skills necessary to practice in these settings; however, site visits revealed that medical schools tended to use managed care settings for teaching because they were good clinical sites with large patient bases, rather than because of the unique managed care experience they offer.

Survey responses suggest that the evolution of managed care in the inner city is gradually affecting medical teaching. Although responding hospitals reported that market forces, especially managed care, do affect these programs, broad changes in the graduate medical education are just becoming evident. The challenge is balancing AHCs' historical core emphasis on specialty care when the need in the community is clearly for primary care training. Training programs must be reorganized to adjust academic goals to the structural demands of managed care organizations. The survey found that the increased need for primary care physicians does influence residency training programs. To meet the demands of managed care plans AHCs must both recognize and operationalize that need and begin to shift their focus from training specialists to training primary care providers (Friedman, 1997b). In the survey, 70 percent of respondents confirmed this contention. This shift of clinical medicine from hospital- to community-based care, with concomitant shifts in training, is not new. It has been heralded as necessary for at least ten years (Friedman, 1997b). Apparently AHCs have been slow to accept or have had difficulty in taking this step.

The survey documented the occurrence of residency shifts in specialty areas. Responding urban-based hospitals have a ratio of three specialists to one primary care physician. Overall, more than 20 percent of the surveyed hospitals decreased their number of specialty positions in several key specialty areas in anesthesiology (39 percent), internal medicine subspecialties (34 percent), pathology (29 percent), and psychiatry (22 percent). In very few cases are training programs going to increase. However, a considerable percentage of reporting hospitals, 31 percent, expects to increase family medicine residencies.

Some professionals have advocated that academic medical settings must take more responsibility for developing and maintaining community-based primary care, social support, and care for isolated and impoverished populations, as well as for furthering knowledge on the broader social and health issues of the disadvantaged. Reorientation of AHCs to such objectives directly complements the mission of public teaching hospitals and represents directions that these hospitals must take to survive (Foreman, 1994).

In all, these changes will not come easily. Academic medicine may be its own worst enemy: the traditional inertia of academic medicine may impede critical curriculum changes that link public health and more traditional training (Their, 1994). This inertia may explain why several public teaching hospitals affiliated with prestigious AHCs (for example, Parkland in Dallas) have decided to take their fate into their own hands by taking such actions as employing their own primary care physicians independent of the medical school (Andrulis, Acuff, Weiss, and Anderson, 1996).

Impact on Research and Specialty Programs

Growing concern also surrounds the fate of research and specialty programs in urban settings. AHCs conduct 42 percent of the health research and development in the United States (Reuter, 1997b). One fear is that managed care and market pressures may reorient research in many teaching hospitals away from vulnerable populations and their conditions. Many managed care organizations are reluctant to provide additional support for research costs incurred by providers and their teaching affiliates. If they do support such activities, they may require research that addresses their own concerns. Although these concerns may coincide with current research priorities, some plans may want to shift focus away from vulnerable populations toward more mainstream enrollees. Alternatively they may choose to stress research on more cost-efficient interventions, to the detriment of therapies that may be more effective but costly. These directions are not inherently conflicting, but at the very least they will need to be reconciled with existing efforts. A darker scenario portends that research areas such as substance abuse and homelessness may give way to other priorities or that managed care will simply offer little support for research at all.

As necessary reorientation of the health system creates greater incentives for primary care, inner-city providers must determine how to sustain essential specialty care services. This is an especially difficult challenge for institutions offering care to inner-city residents, since they may be the only resource for such services. At the same time, these specialty areas may become major financial cost centers, based on the population served and the high price of maintaining such care. For example, trauma care, an essential service in the inner city, may also be very unprofitable due to hospital location, numbers of uninsured treated, and lack of adequate reimbursement.

As primary components of the urban safety net, public teaching hospitals face daunting challenges as they adapt to a competitive marketplace and strive to maintain a mission that focuses on vulnerable populations not only through services in general but also in specialty care. Despite these challenges, many of these institutions see significant opportunity to succeed in this new environment through their historical health care responsibilities, community ties, and strategic redirections. For example, Parkland Hospital in Dallas believes that its reputation as a facility open to all regardless of ability to pay will serve it well, especially since a number of its awards for high-quality service have become known in the community. It is planning to maintain, if not increase, market share through its own HMO. In addition, it is developing a sophisticated set of community-based and public health–related programs, and it is integrating its products to include a range of services from primary care through rehabilitation. Another safety net hospital, Denver Health (DH), sees its community clinics as forming a fundamental part of its core strengths in the Denver area, especially as it continues to develop its managed care strategy. San Francisco General (SFGH) uses its status as one of the premier AIDS providers in the

United States, as well as the largest single provider of the area's inpatient mental health services, to maintain its competitive market position.

Parkland, SFGH, and DH also intend to build on two common characteristics: high volume of ambulatory care and status as "centers of excellence," especially in high-cost or essential services such as trauma and poison control centers. Parkland has developed smaller niche centers of excellence such as an epilepsy center and a transplant center. Parkland is entering into a marketing relationship with several managed care companies to promote these programs. Public teaching hospitals hope that centers of excellence will appeal to commercial insurers, managed care plans contracting for specialty services, and possibly to a regional or national market (Andrulis, Acuff, Weiss, and Anderson, 1996).

Conclusions

Academic medicine and managed care represent important and potentially complementary strengths for the benefits of inner-city residents. Academic medicine's strengths include experience in delivering high-quality care to insured and uninsured individuals and leadership in research and clinical outcomes. Managed care can bring a focus on efficiency and patient satisfaction. Notwithstanding the benefits, teaching hospitals and affiliated medical schools face special challenges in adapting to managed care. These challenges include difficulty in evolving to an integrated delivery system from an acute care orientation, redirecting the focus on specialty training, a need to reorient to a new reimbursement structure not based on fee-for-service, and conflicting intraorganizational objectives related to multiple missions. Most, if not all, teaching hospitals have concluded that their survival and future success lie in redirecting the inpatient focus to primary and community health care.

A service-related concern is the role of specialty care. Many communities undoubtedly will continue to need the specialty care that teaching hospitals provide. Not only will those who cannot afford to pay still depend on these settings, but the broader community will still expect to have access to high-quality essential services such as trauma and burn care services frequently located in these institutions. The ability of AHCs to work successfully with managed care will affect the fate of these services. Further investigation might consider whether AHCs' or hospitals' support for unprofitable services will be reduced or eliminated. Future studies might also consider whether these institutions effectively integrate primary and specialty care.

Finally, all the discourse around efficiency and primary care leaves open to question how to sustain the important research and training activities of inner-city providers. The goals of both managed care and teaching hospitals need recognition in these arenas. Finding common ground becomes imperative if these essential missions are to thrive. Education of future physicians, especially those who will be practicing in a managed care environment in the inner city, will suffer, as will those in need, if the situation of residents—their conditions, diversity, and social circumstances—cannot be reconciled with the course being charted.

Chapter Five

Financing Managed Care
for Urban Populations

By the mid-1990s, all states but Alaska and Wyoming had established some form of Medicaid managed care. These programs cover almost half of the Medicaid enrollment in managed care.

Many reports have documented the benefits from achieving Medicaid eligibility for those who had been uninsured. For example, analysis of data from the National Medical Expenditure Survey and the Survey of Income and Program Participation over time revealed that those uninsured AFDC patients who became eligible for Medicaid significantly increased both ambulatory and inpatient service use, and approached private insurance use rates (Marquis and Long, 1996). In all, access to care for this population is increased through Medicaid eligibility. However, even with the perceived benefits for the uninsured, some access barriers remain since a proportion of beneficiaries are in poorer health and probably use more services. A key conclusion drawn from the research related to Medicaid financing and care for such vulnerable populations is that measures to limit per capita spending might place some of the Medicaid population groups at risk of underservice unless the spending limits account for the differences in the health status and needs of the subpopulations (Marquis and Long, 1996).

Medicaid faces other challenges related to physician participation and the patient population. For example, physician noncompliance, high-risk populations, little primary or preventive care, lack of adequate documentation, high administrative responsibilities, and low reimbursement rates have encumbered the delivery of services or proved a disincentive for physicians to accept Medicaid

patients (Witek and Hostage, 1994). The physician shortage is especially felt in urban areas where there are low numbers of physicians
who accept Medicaid and high numbers of Medicaid beneficiaries.
Many Medicaid recipients are less healthy and less compliant compared to their non-Medicaid counterparts. Nonetheless, this report
indicates that Medicaid managed care patients in this population
had slightly better access to care than did regular fee-for-service
patients.

What do these findings and conclusions about Medicaid expansion mean when they are applied to the inner city? The expansion
of Medicaid in urban areas suggests the potential of substantially
greater access for those who historically have been left out of mainstream health care. Nonetheless, it points to several issues that, if
left unaddressed, threaten to handicap many managed care initiatives in urban settings significantly.

This chapter reviews recent changes in Medicaid and other
financing for health care as they affect residents in the inner city,
provider systems, and managed care. It is not intended to serve as a
summary of the extensive information already available from
numerous sources on Medicaid managed care or other resources.
Instead, it targets several areas of concern for the populations in
need of care and the safety net issues within the inner-city environment. In so doing, it draws lessons and questions from the
broader financing discussions that bring to light implications for
urban populations, managed care, and the safety net.

Reimbursement and Financing in
the Context of the Marketplace

Even as managed care expansion takes place for vulnerable populations and communities generally around the country, health care
programs in a marketplace increasingly sensitive to the bottom line
are beginning to reassess their ability to follow through on an initially promising commitment to Medicaid. An article in the New

York Times ("Largest HMOs . . . ," 1998) found that managed care organizations in at least twelve states have shut down their services related to Medicaid, while others are reducing their involvement with Medicaid. Some of the key reasons have to do with reimbursement rates. The article notes in particular that states with large populations and substantial urban poverty are especially vulnerable.

A 1998 report on the relationship of commercial HMOs and Medicaid using information from the National Association of Insurance Commissioners filings and other sources found a less-than-optimistic scenario among these private managed care companies as well. In particular, pressures resulting from lowering Medicaid rates instituted by states, expanded beneficiary enrollment base, greater contract specification, and doubts over the long-term intentions of states in their relationship with the private HMO market (and a bias toward the existing safety net, many of them still struggling to reorient to managed care) leave many HMO executives skeptical of success. Compounding these concerns is the overall negative perspective of the stock market on managed care ventures into Medicaid. The report recommends that states consider stabilizing rates at an adequate level to create a more promising Medicaid managed care potential. Clarity in contractor qualifications and creation of more cooperative, less adversarial relationships will assist in implementing and sustaining a successful Medicaid managed care effort (Hurley and McCue, 1998).

These findings should raise a cautionary note to inner cities. Many managed care organizations have not reached a firm conclusion about the viability of their programs for low-income communities and individuals. At the very least, this assessment is continuing and may result in additional exits of plans. In a more dire scenario, without sufficient financial support and shared responsibility, these difficult urban areas may be left with fragmented, fragile managed care programs unable to meet the demands of a long-neglected population.

Capitation Rates, Risk Adjustment, and Adverse Selection

The determination of payment based on population characteristics is central to the viability of any implemented managed care program. For inner-city providers, the extent to which capitation rates capture health and health-related needs will spell the difference between effective, sustained provider participation, incorporating the spectrum of required services, and restrictive care or nonparticipation.

A 1995 study compared cost data for commercial and Medicaid enrollees from nine HMOs (Welch and Wade, 1995). As a point of comparison, it measured the ratio of the cost per member per month of Medicaid mothers and children and commercial enrollees. Results from the analysis determined that costs per Medicaid enrollee generally were 13 percent higher than the average commercial enrollee. Conclusions suggest that Medicaid HMO premiums should be set at 113 percent of commercial premiums to cover the difference in costs. Utilization of a Colorado Kaiser HMO by previously uninsured individuals with incomes up to 200 percent of poverty revealed similar patterns to those of a control group of new commercial enrollees, at moderately greater costs (Bograd and others, 1997). Ambulatory visits were found to be substantially higher among the previously uninsured, but the higher-cost services related to inpatient care, as well as pharmacy, tests, and radiology, were not significantly different. The authors determined that the "results did not support the hypothesis that greater pent-up demand for services in the previously uninsured study group would lead to their having a more intense start-up effect than the control group" (Bograd and others, 1997, p. 1070).

Nonetheless, since greater intensity of use might have been expected among the uninsured, the authors suggest that noninsurance barriers such as transportation, time available, and overall perceived value of health care by patients may have limited utilization. However, they conclude that financial costs may decrease once stability in enrollment is achieved. In all, the authors suggest that "uninsured groups can be served within managed care settings at only moderately more cost than that required for commercial group" (Bograd and others, 1997, p. 1072). In all, these studies support the contention that additional but not exorbitant costs should be expected in caring for these populations. State Medicaid programs and other financing entities should be prepared to adjust payments for these costs.

Adverse selection also represents a potentially significant financial threat. Adverse selection problems for plans or providers that are plan affiliates can arise in at least two ways: (1) an urban managed care plan assumes responsibility for an inner-city area in which enrollees have disproportionately high rates of difficult-to-treat and high-cost problems (such as violence-related trauma, combined with high rates of substance abuse and chronic conditions); or (2) a provider or plan encounters a population pocket of high-cost enrollees such as low-income individuals with HIV. Either of these scenarios will create financial difficulties at the very least and could eventually threaten solvency. Alternatively, managed care organizations will be tempted to screen out or somehow "red-line" those individuals and areas that are likely to cost more.

Appropriate risk- and population-related payment adjustments would alleviate this problem, because plans would have sufficient funding to care for these individuals, and other plans or providers may be less reluctant to take on higher-cost individuals. In these cases, the financing entities (employers and local and state Medicaid managed care programs in particular) will need to recognize and adjust for this selection. Maryland has recently instituted risk adjustments to account for these circumstances. Some states have plans assume risk for some portion of medical expenses; however, the plans are not fully capitated. Other payers are using a stop-loss plan that seems to be effective with low-income mothers and their children; less progress has occurred with SSI recipients.

Finally, one of the concerns that professionals in managed care express is that if they are effective at serving populations that are difficult to treat, the providers or plans will become magnets for many more, thus limiting their ability to expand toward more mainstream enrollees and hurting their bottom line. For example, Oxford Health Plan in New York City found that because it was doing so well managing the Medicaid population, it started seeing a disproportionate share of high-risk patients with lower capitation rates. Others, such as Humana, have concluded that they could provide care when Medicaid payments were in proportion to treatment delivered, but could not afford to have an excessive proportion of Medicaid enrollees. From the provider perspective, if a physician establishes a practice in the inner city, people will come regardless of their ability to pay. Without sufficient numbers of providers to spread the financial risk, those who stay may be saddled with both lower capitation rates and high numbers of uninsured patients.

The Challenge of Attaining Stability in Enrollment

Perhaps one of the most challenging financial issues facing managed care is the cyclical or episodic nature of Medicaid eligibility. This on again–off again shifting status leaves plans unable to predict their caseload, financial reimbursement, and overall service demand.

Changes in welfare threaten to complicate eligibility problems even further. Early review of welfare and immigration reforms suggested that the sudden declines in government assistance programs (welfare rolls fell 26 percent between 1993 and 1997, from 14 million to 10.5 million) are having a perhaps serious side effect of reducing Medicaid numbers as well (Ellwood and Ku, 1998).

This phenomenon affects financing and service objectives in managed care organizations, encumbering provider or plan ability to fulfill obligations to enrollees and reducing their responsibilities to those enrollees. Variable eligibility hinders continuity of care substantially. Short enrollment periods lead to an acute episodic care environment rather than a health maintenance environment, which can refocus health care more positively and ultimately lead

to cost savings. For the managed care organization, short enrollment periods discourage investments in the health of the enrolled
populations. Consequently the benefit of investing in the long-term
well-being of individuals cannot be realized.

In order to be effective, managed care needs adequate financial
and enrollment stability for the provider and the plan. In the ab-
sence of that stability, a downward spiral may occur. For example,
in some Medicaid managed care programs, payment rates begin at
an adequate level for a certain number of enrollees when based on
a fee-for-service equivalent; however, over time states may reduce
those rates. This situation makes it more difficult for a plan to be
financially viable.

Although there is no single solution to the problem of episodic
eligibility, the situation may be improved through targeted initiatives such as mandating enrollee lock-in and sharing information
and records among institutions with a history of treating inner-city
patients. Achieving this consistency and experience also will help
enrollees by giving them a chance to learn the system and by providing a longer-term provider relationship. In some cases, for example, at Denver Health, the public provider system sustains plan
membership for some period even if an enrollee loses Medicaid. In
other cases, managed care organizations can work to sustain eligibility by assisting in the completion of documentation, notifying
recipients when they need to reapply, and becoming advocates for
ensuring their eligibility.

Another strategy for sustaining enrollment levels is a default
assignment methodology to traditional providers of care for Medicaid recipients who do not enroll in a plan. Although Medicaid
managed care is required to offer some choice of plans to enrollees,
many individuals either do not select a plan when completing forms
or do not register for a specific plan. In these cases eligible beneficiaries are automatically assigned, or defaulted, into a plan that is
designated under contract. The United Health Plan of Los Angeles
has estimated that delays in default plan guidelines by the state of

California cost it $25 million in lost revenues, based on the assumption that a large portion of the eligible population would not complete the designated provider process.

Such revenues, important for any plan, are critical to managed care plans sponsored by safety net organizations. The importance to safety net providers is that the Medicaid population is a traditional source of customers and revenues. Given the highlighted competition, however, Medicaid patients now are attractive to other organizations. In many cases, the ability of safety net plans and providers to continue to capture this revenue may make the difference between effective organizational transition and success, and inability to maintain a payment base sufficient for survival.

The federally enacted State Child Health Insurance Program represents a nexus of enrollment and financing challenges and opportunities for managed care and affiliated providers. This initiative provides an infusion of federal and state matching funds to states to expand their coverage of children. Coverage may be provided by either the state's Medicaid program or a separate program. Managed care and other providers may find that it is in their best interest to assist, if not become active advocates for beneficiaries, in the enrollment process. In particular, it may make sense for them to work to ensure seamless coverage either within the Medicaid program or for those who may alternate eligibility between Medicaid and a state-only child health initiative. This seamlessness will enable beneficiaries to continue to participate in a plan even if their eligibility status changes.

The Special Circumstances of the Uninsured

An article in the New York Times ("Government Lags . . . ," 1998) refocused attention on the fact that over 41 million individuals are uninsured, a number that has increased yearly since 1987. Yet discussions focusing on managed care frequently sidestep the problems of individuals who, for a variety of reasons, are not enrolled in any publicly or privately financed insurance program. In the nation's inner cities, these individuals are diverse and include many working-poor families who do not qualify for assistance, for example immigrants and single men and women. Moreover, Weissman (1996) has noted that not only are the uninsured as a proportion of the population increasing, but the underinsured (those who have difficulty meeting the medical costs they incur) have increased approximately 50 percent since the mid-1980s, to represent 25 to 48 million additional individuals. Reasons for concern that these numbers will continue to increase include the decline in the number of persons covered by employer-based insurance (especially difficult for inner-city populations in the light of welfare-to-work initiatives and the likelihood of employment in service sector positions); the likelihood that most Medicaid waiver programs will not cover all uninsured; and the fact that Medicaid expansion does not guarantee payment adequacy. For example, assessment of early Tenncare experiences found that Medicaid payment rates were 40 percent below actuarial soundness.

To date, cross-subsidization, or using the revenues generated from certain paying patients to cover the costs of those with insufficient funds to pay for care, has been a major source of support on which public and private health care organizations have relied to cover the costs of their services. The individuals who depend on these providers and their resources are already at a significant disadvantage as measured by access to care. For example, one study that used the 1980 National Medical Care Expenditure Survey data found that the uninsured used substantially fewer ambulatory and inpatient care resources compared with those who were privately insured (Spillman, 1992). In general, the increasing influence of managed care threatens to create additional financial barriers for those without insurance. However, in the inner city, the situation may be more acute due to concentrations of poverty and complex social and health conditions. Thus, inner-city health care providers who attempt to incorporate indigent care into their capitation rate estimates may be outbid by other organizations that treat significantly fewer people who cannot pay. In this case, managed care plans may leave these service providers with limited and unpleasant choices: incur greater proportional losses; seek assistance from other sources, if available; or curtail services to this population.

To date, the traditional providers of indigent care have attempted to maintain their level of financial support even though the proportion of care for the uninsured is increasing (or related revenues are declining, or both) for many community health centers, safety net hospitals, and similar organizations. Nonetheless, the cost and enrollee restrictions applied by managed care plans may clarify the choice for their current or potential provider affiliates: reduce indigent care or lose their contracts. One conclusion regarding the tightening financial picture propelled by managed care and cost containment is that "continued expansion of managed care for persons with public and private coverage remains on a potential collision course with the cost-shifting that finances much of the uncompensated care in this country" (Hurley and Walin, 1998, p. 24).

The Threat and the Opportunity for
Inner-City Safety Net Hospitals

The issues concerning higher-risk, higher-cost enrollees are confronting inner-city safety net hospitals that are striving to adapt to managed care in two major ways. First, the sheer number of uninsured individuals and those with difficult-to-treat conditions result in the need to generate sufficient revenues through cross-subsidies and government sources. This need places safety net institutions at a competitive disadvantage in negotiations with managed care plans. A frequently omitted fact in health care expansion discussions is that millions of low-income single men and women will not qualify for any insurance program and will remain dependent on the safety net. Second, many inner-city safety net providers, in particular teaching hospitals, face organizational barriers in adapting quickly to the new managerial, informational, and structural demands (for example, by reorientation to outpatient and community-based care). In the fast-moving arena of the current marketplace, such difficulty also places these providers at a significant disadvantage.

In their search for financial resources to assist in the transition to managed care and to offset the high costs of their populations, many inner-city safety net hospitals rely on support in the form of disproportionate share hospital (DSH) payments through Medicaid; these are special add-on Medicaid payments to hospitals serving large numbers of low-income patients. The future of such support is far from clear. A review of uncompensated hospital care cited the American Hospital Association's estimate of an annual average of $16 billion in costs (Weissman, 1996). DSH support rose from $1 billion in 1989 to $15 billion in 1997. (These payments were capped after Congress determined that not all funds were being used for health care.) DSH funds are one of the primary sources by which hospitals have offset indigent care costs, frequently supplementing state and local monies that are used to assist in the transition to managed care. However, many state Medicaid programs (Tenncare is one of them) are incorporating this support into their waiver-based initiatives. In so doing, the guarantee of continued DSH to the hospitals is being replaced by uncertainty, dilution, or elimination of such support. Thus, in addition to the competitive disadvantage facing these providers by the nature of their mission, redirection may further encumber the hospitals' ability to maintain their commitments to these populations and, in some circumstances, even to survive.

Although many inner-city providers have felt increasingly constrained by the limited and generally difficult alternatives facing them, several health care organizations with community obligations to care for those without insurance have worked with their state and local governments to create opportunity to improve the care to their vulnerable populations by incorporating indigent enrollees into managed care. In particular, public hospital systems in inner cities, frequently in conjunction with their counties, have designed managed care programs. Some examples of these systems follow.

Contra Costa Health Plan (CCHP), Contra Costa, California. CCHP was the first public HMO to become federally qualified. Established in 1973, it is part of the county Health Services Department. The plan, owned and operated by the county, is open to all Medi-Cal groups, Medicare beneficiaries, indigent beneficiaries covered under the basic adult care program, and individuals with private insurance. The 1998 enrollment was 49,790 individuals; 75 percent of the enrollment is covered by Medi-Cal. To encourage enrollment, the plan offers twenty-four-hour access to health care providers. The provider network includes approximately forty-two primary care physicians and twenty-two specialty physicians and the county hospital. The county also contracts with other hospitals for tertiary care.

Jackson Memorial Health Plan (JMHHP), Miami, Florida. JMHHP was established in 1985 in Dade County, Florida, as a state plan–defined HMO. It is organized as a department within Jackson Memorial Hospital. The plan, which enrolls Medicaid recipients on a voluntary basis, is open to all Medicaid-eligible as well as private-pay clients. To encourage enrollment, the plan waives copayments and offers special education programs. The current enrollment is 5,700 county employees, 5,400 children covered under the Healthy Kids program, and 21,700 Medicaid enrollees. The network includes university and community-based PCPs (primary care practitioners), specialists, and hospitals. The plan contracts with the University of Miami School of Medicine for specialty referral services.

Metropolitan Health Plan (MHP), Minneapolis, Minnesota. MHP was established in 1983 under a Section 1115 demonstration waiver (in federal statutes). Because the Minnesota Medicaid program is administered at the county level, the state Medicaid agency initiated several county-based managed care demonstration projects, including MHP. Located in Hennepin County, the HMO is owned and operated by the county, and it is organized within the county's Bureau of Health. It has no separate corporate identity.

MHP enrolls Medical Assistance (GMAC) recipients, a state-funded program for low-income individuals and county employees. In Hennepin County, enrollment in managed care plans is mandatory for all Medical Assistance and GMAC recipients, with a twelve-month lock-in period. MHP competes with three other managed care plans. As of August 1998, plan enrollment was 27,000.

Wishard Advantage—Indianapolis, Indiana. The Health and Hospital Corporation (which operates Wishard Health Services and the Indiana University School of Medicine, and oversees the university physicians) developed a joint primary care initiative known as Indiana Health Care, Inc. (IHC). One of IHC's projects is a managed care program for low-income patients. The program, Wishard Advantage, operates much like commercial or Medicaid managed care insurance plans and is one of a handful of programs in the nation to apply managed care concepts to an uninsured population.

Wishard Advantage is a managed care program that is open to Marion County residents and their families who are at or below 200 percent of the federal poverty level. Wishard Advantage is a health-cost assistance program, not an insurance plan. Only services provided by its network providers are covered; care received outside the network is not reimbursed.

Wishard Advantage operates like other managed care programs. All qualifying low-income patients and their family members who receive care in the Wishard Health Services delivery system either choose or are assigned a primary care physician.

All of these initiatives share a number of common elements. They have at least minimally sufficient financial support from either governmental sources alone or in combination with other venues (such as foundations); they seek to capitalize on the emerging or traditional strengths of the organizations such as clinic networks; and they are consonant with the organizational missions. These programs are not simple short-lived experiments. Rather, they were put in place to address a chronic problem of access to care for populations historically and recently passed over in the implementation of managed care.

Conclusion

Government and private purchasers have vested managed care with the power to control and direct their dollars. In so doing, these organizations have placed new and significant demands on providers in the inner city and elsewhere to reduce costs, become more efficient, and be accountable for financing care and patient outcomes.

By turning to managed care through the use of Medicaid waivers, several states have sought an opportunity to expand coverage for the previously uninsured. This expansion, at least in the short run, may improve financial access for some inner-city residents. However, long-standing issues in reimbursement generally and specifically related to managed care may significantly encumber, if not thwart the success of, caring for those in the nation's cities by discouraging broader provider responsibility and encumbering those willing to care for difficult to treat populations. Following are the major concerns:

- Inadequate Medicaid payments and unproductive relationships between states and managed care organizations

- Inadequate capitation, rates, and risk adjustment to account for the complexity and historical neglect typical of many inner-city communities

- Adverse selection of high-cost or complex cases for managed care plans and their providers based on location, mission to serve the underserved, or other circumstances

- Difficulties in attaining stability in enrollment and financing as urban residents experience cyclical eligibility, a situation that undermines the fundamental features, as well as incentive for managed care to invest in the health of individuals for the long term

- Cost and consequences to those treating large numbers of uninsured, especially as alternatives for payment such as cross subsidization are reduced or phased out altogether

Notwithstanding the discussions regarding their role, inner-city safety net hospitals and health centers may collectively be the most vulnerable providers. Whereas other health care organizations may consider expansion into marketing to increase Medicaid enrollment an entrepreneurial venture, this paying patient group represents the lifeblood of many safety net providers. Without this population, many would not survive due to their higher volumes of uninsured and those such as substance-dependent persons who are difficult to treat. Greatly reduced capacity to cross-subsidize care to the uninsured, questionable future targeting of disproportionate share support, and lower government financing for the poor aggravate the situation. Finally, although some public sources have been successfully applied to develop managed care for the uninsured, without recognition of the vulnerable population costs, something will likely have to give—and that may result in forced reduced commitment to the neediest inner-city residents or an abrogation of safety net mission. Alternatively, many of these safety net organizations have demonstrated over time a remarkable ability to survive and adapt to the changing financial environments without severely compromising their mission. With financial recognition of what is needed to sustain them, they could become effective collaborators with managed care in designing a greatly improved health care system for the inner city.

Chapter Six

Toward an Effective Managed Care System for the Nation's Inner Cities

To date, the inner city and its residents' health care needs have not been the focus of attention in planning the future of managed care. Nonetheless, the dynamics around managed care—state Medicaid changes, regulatory activities, alliances, and other public or private actions—are affecting these communities. In addition, the traditional providers of care remain a central part of this unfolding scenario. In all, the formative environment around managed care presents opportunities for significant positive effect in these communities.

As we examine selected or recommended actions and place them in the context of the inner city, we describe some of the important initiatives at the state level, the role of the private sector, and implications for populations and the urban safety net. We also discuss state and federal actions to guide managed care and identify eight policy priorities based on the information and review presented in this book. These are intended to assist inner-city communities in creating cost-effective managed care systems. A closing recommendation warns of the likelihood of failure to improve health in the inner city without resolution among managed care and affiliated providers to incorporate the community environment that so significantly influences health into the mission of promoting health and preventing illness.

The Actions of Government in Service and Financing Policy

Government at all levels has stepped into the managed care arena by taking the lead in establishing policies affecting urban residents and their health care providers. Led by the devolution of increasing responsibility for health and social services from federal to state government, states have used their new-found authority to undertake changes through Medicaid waivers and other programs.

State Policies, Medicaid Reform, and the Effect on Inner-City Providers

Responsibilities and resources for the shaping of health care for vulnerable populations have largely been transferred from Washington to the states and thus have provided states with the opportunity to reshape their provider systems generally and especially their safety net. We briefly describe how a number of states have chosen to use this authority and the early indications of effects on populations of concern.

According to a 1997 report from the Urban Institute, a research organization, the safety net in Washington State in urban areas and beyond seems to be in a strong position for continuing its role for vulnerable populations in the era of managed care (Nichols, Ku, Norton, and Wall, 1997). This status has been achieved for a number of reasons. In the Seattle area, the two major safety net hospital systems, Harborview Medical Center and Children's Hospital, have capitalized on their status as preeminent providers of high-quality specialty care (trauma and certain tertiary care for Harborview, and pediatric care for Children's). The disproportionate share program also remains strong, with the state using the funds to target safety net providers such as Harborview. In addition, community health centers have been able to position themselves for competition through creating their own provider network that can bid for capitated contracts. These providers have become more cost-effective by developing promising networks and affiliations, and they have better managed their resources. The state's program also allows safety net–based and other plans to keep the savings they accrue from capitation. Local health departments have oriented services toward broader community health issues such as promoting health and conducting assessments. Nonetheless, strong competition and overbedding loom as factors that can upset the currently healthy status of these providers.

Another Urban Institute report considered the changes in health policy in Minnesota (Coughlin, Rajan, Zuckerman, and Marstellar, 1997). That state operates two major programs for low-income populations, one initiated through a Section 1115 Medicaid waiver project (the Prepaid Medical Assistance Project) and a state program for uninsured individuals and families with children not otherwise covered (MinnesotaCare), which has been operating since 1992 and insures over 100,000 individuals. Although the state has considerable experience with managed care and has been working to develop its programs for low-income populations for some time, the fate of the safety net has become more uncertain. Concern among urban and rural counties has heightened because of the perceived threat that the Medicaid 1115 waivers, the Prepaid Medical Assistance Project, would lead to a significantly lessened role for them and their health departments. This resulted in a requirement that counties must approve this program when it enters a new area. In part, this may be reflective of the county concern that service costs could be shifted down to them from the state. At the same time, the state has attempted to encourage health departments to move away from direct services to environmental health and health promotion.

As in Washington State, community health centers in Minnesota have been developing their own networks to gain greater advantage in negotiating with managed care organizations, create a broader base of support, and become more efficient. The Urban Institute report concludes that the future of these centers, which are a critical resource in Minneapolis, may be threatened due to an intended state phase-out of cost-based reimbursement in a few years. At the same time, the state has agreed to assist centers through a three-year transition period so that such reimbursement can continue for those three years. Urban safety net hospitals such as Hennepin County Medical Center in Minneapolis are seeking ways to reduce costs. Although the uncompensated care rate is comparatively low, managed care penetration is forcing hospitals in general to accept lower payment rates. In addition, the Medicaid admission distribution under managed care is broadening the locus of inpatient care beyond the traditional providers so that the city's public hospital may face a reduction in a key source of payment. DSH payments under Medicaid managed care were also folded into plans' capitation rates.

Notwithstanding these provider issues, recent research has confirmed that the program for non-Medicaid-eligible individuals seems to be having some positive effect. A survey-based report on the first years of the MinnesotaCare program (1990–1995) was completed in 1997 (Theide and others, 1997). Although the program is acknowledged as being far from perfect, the report documented that MinnesotaCare contributed to a sustained low rate of uninsurance and a reduction in the number of uninsured children. Moreover, the study did not confirm fears that the program would supplant the private insurance employment-based market.

In an action that extended beyond Medicaid, the state of Michigan established CountyCare as a managed care alternative for the non-Medicaid poor (Douglass and Torres, 1994). Providers participating in this program receive seventy dollars per member per month, and patients who present themselves at locations that are not part of their member networks are triaged back to the institutions in an attempt to prevent out-of-program utilization.

A related survey examined service utilization and patient satisfaction for an urban indigent population participating in a managed care system with multiple providers, serving primarily general assistance recipients who were older, generally male African American, and without dependent children (Douglass and Torres, 1994). Respondents reported a high level of utilization of services and the pharmacy, and just over half reported that the managed care system was a good medical care system. The authors found that the enrollees in CountyCare used the managed care services in addition to, not instead of, the usual sources of care. One of the conclusions is that the medically indigent do not respond to managed care as well as others who may be more aware of the financial components associated with the program.

These examples point out the variability of effect and the safety net response to state actions. They demonstrate both benefits that can accrue from these actions and the uncertainty left by the current environment.

Underlying these profiles are important trends reflecting at least three critical and unresolved policy questions. First, how can states find the balance between supporting expansion of eligibility and services to low-income populations on the one hand, and assisting or protecting the traditional safety net providers? To leave this group without help at least in the transition to managed care could not only cripple essential parts of the community delivery system; it could handicap the development of effective managed care systems in such areas as the inner city. Alternatively, a state might significantly decrease its number of uninsured and expand financial access to care by applying the Medicaid Disproportionate Share Adjustment funds (additional support through Medicaid for providers caring for large numbers of poor) or other resources to expand Medicaid coverage. Second, what is the optimal mix of safety net and other organizations for populations that are disenfranchised or low income? States are not yet clear on how much their vision of their system will represent a seamlessness wherein Medicaid enrollees will have access to health care regardless of who is providing that care. Finally, what do the changes mean for the uninsured and others who may remain outside any mainstream-funded system? If local changes yield a significantly diminished safety net, then the remaining providers must shoulder responsibility. Such a resolution is difficult to guarantee at a time of increasing financing constriction among public and private providers.

Actions to Regulate Managed Care

A diffuse but dramatic reaction to rein in managed care has followed the relatively recent rush to embrace managed care strategies. By the mid-1990s, a thousand legislative proposals to curtail HMOs in some way had been introduced by state legislatures (Bodenheimer, 1995). One of the initiative areas was access to care, particularly for such vulnerable populations as people with AIDS. Concern was that gatekeeping primary care physicians had less adequate training than infectious disease physicians in caring for these individuals. Curbing limits on emergency department denials also has garnered attention, as have cultural competence–related requirements. Concern continues regarding point-of-service plans being marketed to the more affluent while not being available to those who are enrolled in Medicaid managed care plans.

A New York Times article ("In Medicine, Government Rises Again," 1997) captured in its story headline the change in attitude toward the government's role. It describes how after the debacle of health care reform, where the private sector was seen as the appropriate place for health care system decisions, anecdotal but dramatic denials of care by HMOs, policies limiting a new mother's stay in the hospital by these organizations, and other actions seen as encumbering the doctor-patient relationship have given rise to calls for state or federal government action. Although these actions have emerged as managed care takes hold, they have lacked any coherent direction, although this situation may be changing to some degree due to the emphasis on patient rights (for example, the consideration of a patient bill of rights at the federal level) and quality of care.

While states and the federal government struggle to discern when regulatory or other intervention is required, some evolving actions on the part of managed care organizations could force further control, especially in the context of financial levels of support. Of particular concern are decisions being made by plans that curtail health care access for Medicaid-eligible populations in urban areas and elsewhere. For example, in February 1998 Oxford Health

Plans withdrew from participation in the Connecticut Medicaid program, citing its enrollee financial losses due to reimbursement reductions by the state ("Largest HMOs Cutting the Poor . . . ," 1998). Oxford has also dropped coverage of New Jersey Medicaid enrollees. A New York Legal Aid Society attorney commented that "the state should not allow plans to come and go as if what they were doing was selling furniture, not health care," voicing concern over continued participation by Oxford in New York. New York had already lost US Healthcare in January 1998, while some plans are even reconsidering their involvement with Medicare, a historically better payer than Medicaid. If similar actions occur in other cities and states, they would threaten to leave the poor (and elderly) out of mainstream managed care. It may also expose states to additional difficulties in ensuring access to quality care and creating the all-important enrollee-provider relationship.

Access, Managed Care, and the Role of the Private Sector

Clearly, many private health care organizations are also dedicated to objectives similar to traditional safety net providers. However, some professionals have argued that in its rapid expansion, managed care threatens to address health far too narrowly, thereby focusing its mission and accountability on its immediate population (Showstack and others, 1996). They challenge managed care organizations in particular to assume a broader community-level responsibility that includes eight areas of social responsibility:

- Enrolling a proportionate representation that cuts across socioeconomic lines
- Assisting and participating collaboratively in initiatives to improve a community's health
- Participating in data network development and data sharing to form a community health information system
- Releasing information on community contribution and financial performance as they relate to the community

- Including broad representation of both traditional and historically marginalized groups in its advisory and governance

- Support and participation in health professions education,
  especially in collaboration with academic health centers

- Working to guarantee a viable public health infrastructure
  by collaborating with key groups such as health departments

- Advocating for community programs in health promotion
  and disease prevention

The private sector also can assist by applying health tracking
and measurement more broadly to cover community health.

Policy Directions for Creating a
High-Quality Managed Care System

Forging effective directions in an arena as complex as the nation's
inner cities is daunting. Divesting of much responsibility by the federal government to the states as well as diverse state policies create
an atmosphere of great turgidity, if not ambiguity. Added to this mix
are the uncertainties—and some disillusionment—around managed care and its capacity to create a cost-effective health care system throughout the United States.

As with the rapidly decreasing fee-for-service approach to health
care, managed care will never be the answer that Americans have
been waiting for. In fact, in its short period of rapid expansion, it has
begun to mutate, forming variations to accommodate to markets.
What its evolution will lead to in ten or twenty years is uncertain.

At the same time, managed care in its various forms is a dom-
inant trend that provides opportunities for the inner city and its
residents. We suggest several areas where policies can assist in developing and sustaining effective inner-city managed care systems
and where safeguards should be put in place to prevent an unrav-
eling of the existing safety net for the protection of these communities.

Supporting Policies Promoting Managed Care Principles
of Greatest Benefit to the Inner City

Many of managed care's fundamentals could bring significant benefit to inner-city residents. Its organizational ability to coordinate services and bring order to what can be a fairly chaotic and diffused system is critical to populations where emergency departments frequently have been the single point of entry. This ability also extends cost efficiencies and rationalizes the delivery systems. Managed care rewards providers for keeping populations healthy. Therefore, managed care can lend much more fiscal responsibility to urban providers of care for the poor. In so doing, it will make primary care a core of any set of services.

Bringing these principles to action in the inner city, where vulnerable populations in particular have suffered from lack of access to ordered, mainstream medical care, is almost radical in its potential impact and meaning. State and local managed care policies, both public and private, should work to nurture these features as they play out in the difficult arena of the nation's inner cities. Policymakers will need to support actions that allow for the complex circumstances of system restructuring in these settings. These actions must incorporate a measured assessment of the role that traditional safety net providers can play—whether full partnerships in public-private affiliations or a more tailored status—and what assistance they will need to be successful in that role. These assessments will need to be balanced with the potential to expand Medicaid eligibility through application of public resources.

Managed Care's Challenge: Adapting to the
Complexities of Factors and Organizations
That Influence Inner-City Health and Health Care

The success of managed care in the nation's cities could bring substantial benefit to its residents; nevertheless, fundamental questions persist about how well many plans fit with the characteristics of the populations, the nature of their needs, and the role of the community. Are managed care plans truly prepared to adapt their ways of doing business to address the complex social and health conditions affecting residents, as well as the reality that improving an enrollee's health is intimately linked to broader community health? Will managed care organizations that have limited experience with the inner city be sufficiently flexible to accommodate the health care preferences of enrollees from different linguistic and cultural backgrounds?

Managed care functions essentially as a closed system, wherein providers are either in or out. In the inner city, many plans will need a more open orientation that includes not only traditional health care providers but also other community institutions: schools, churches, social services, and police. Finally, plans may need to shift in a similar way, incorporating a wider set of disciplines, among them case managers who will be at the core of many service programs.

Promoting Policies That Adjust for Key Factors Most Likely to Affect Provider Financing of Care for Inner-City Residents

Managed care financing methods for urban areas should be developed with special consideration for the additional effort required for inner-city populations. This consideration should include careful structuring of case mix adjustment to incorporate both the complexity of conditions where applicable, and certain so-called wrap-around services, such as language, transportation, nutrition, and social support that may be essential to successful disease-prevention and health interventions. State and local policies also should weigh the potential value of sustaining safety net providers in the inner city during the transition to managed care, especially if the health delivery infrastructure is threatened by closures, elimination of care for the uninsured, and loss of essential community services.

The Relationship of Managed Care and the Safety Net in the Inner City: Striving to Keep the Balance Between Financial Realities and Community and Enrollee Needs

Clearly the revolution created by managed care already has encouraged inner-city safety net providers to become more fiscally efficient and to be recast as part of a system of care. But what happens to providers that do not fit within the marketplace strategy that so dominates current thinking due to their overriding mission to care for vulnerable populations? And what happens to the set of essential community services that are financially costly to maintain and deliver? Does managed care assume no responsibility for trauma care, burn, neonatal intensive care, public health surveillance, and other services—all so critical to the population in the entire area—which could be crippled without sharing of related costs and responsibilities? Ultimately broader coalitions that include providers, community and government representatives, and business, along with managed care organizations, will be necessary to maintain critical features of the inner-city safety net.

Determining U.S. Policy and Managed Care Responsibility for the Uninsured in Cities

The expanded use of Medicaid managed care has made care to the eligible populations attractive to a broader number of providers and managed care plans. But what about those who do not qualify for either public or private insurance? What becomes of them, and what responsibility should managed care-related organizations assume? In the end, managed care plans may find providers of care to this population less attractive and work to eliminate cross-subsidies for support of such care by penalizing those who continue to treat the uninsured. If most managed care plans do not assume a responsibility for these populations and those who care for them, then resources should be adapted to account for the providers and plans. Internal policies or those put forth by government–private sector coalitions should encourage broader shared responsibility, perhaps from the perspective of assuming involvement for the greater community's health.

Directed Regulatory Managed Care Policy at the State and Federal Levels to Safeguard Key Populations in the Inner City

Governments are beginning to structure their efforts to guide managed care. All participants—plans, providers, and inner-city communities—stand to benefit from a more carefully structured regulatory role. For example, states or the federal government, or both, may need to provide assurance to enrollees that their plans will not drop participation for certain periods. In other situations, attention to cultural diversity in training and determination of appropriate support services (such as interpretation) will be critical. Cooperative efforts among concerned entities—government, enrollee advocates especially for Medicaid, managed care plans, and participating providers—such as an advisory body, could assist in bringing issues to attention before they reach the stage where narrow regulatory intervention is seen as necessary.

The Joint Responsibility of Urban Teaching Hospitals and Managed Care

Managed care and urban teaching hospitals must reach agreement on how best to support the service, teaching, and research activities that constitute the mission of these institutions. This does not imply a simple perpetuation of the status quo. On the contrary, these teaching hospitals and their affiliated medical schools must accelerate their adaptation to managed care and to community needs that extend beyond the specialty or inpatient unit. Although many of these education institutions have made strides in creating more responsive organizations, a large number must still close two major gaps they have contributed to creating: their distance from the community they serve and the failure of many to incorporate managed care into their curricula. Failure by organizations to address such core issues may very well place them on the periphery of health system change.

At the same time, managed care must not turn its back on the essential activities that traverse all three mission areas. These organizations represent future providers and play a role in establishing high-quality care for communities. For inner cities, they also deliver a broad spectrum of services to large numbers of low-income and uninsured patients. Managed care must realize that by working constructively with these organizations, they are investing in a community's future and the future of health professions locally and nationally, with a payoff that returns to these plans as well.

Intervention to Improve the Health of America's Cities: The Critical Policy Ingredient for Success in Managed Care

A major review of health conditions in urban areas cited several policy issues that are critical to improving the health of inner-city residents (Freundberg, 1997) and clearly transcend the narrower focus that often occurs in discussions of health care in cities. Instead, this review stresses broader strategies and challenges:

- Reorienting health care policy away from the categorical to more comprehensive approaches
- The need for more effective communication across agencies and systems to address the broader problems of drug abuse, infant mortality, and homelessness
- The need to create conjoint efforts traversing all levels of government
- The need to move beyond the individual level to institutional and policy change

A 1997 assessment of a multiyear program to provide comprehensive assistance to young, disadvantaged mothers provides dramatic evidence of what happens when the best-intentioned efforts fail to incorporate this broader level into their intervention. The New York City–based Manpower Development Research Corporation had implemented a sixteen-site, ten-state demonstration specifically intended to break the cycle of welfare dependency, unemployment, and repeated pregnancy that plagues many young, low-income women. The demonstration attempted to accomplish this change through more intensive education, career and job placement, parenting and family planning, and other actions (Quint, Bos, and Polit, 1997).

The general conclusion was that after three and one-half years, the demonstration had not succeeded: the great majority of the experimental group remained both poor and on welfare; the experimental group showed little difference from the control group by measures of pregnancies, births, and abortions; and children's preschool readiness did not improve significantly. In addition, women in the experimental group were found to be slightly but significantly more depressed, suggesting that the program increased hopeful expectations of change in their lives that did not occur. Finally, both the experimental and control group women expressed initial interest in education, but several factors inhibited the sustaining of interest over time—homelessness, violence in the home, inadequate transportation and child care, and health concerns—which become exacerbated over the contention on the part of the women that their employment will separate them from the safety net by eliminating their public insurance coverage. In capturing the broad set of factors that affect the outcome, the report recommends that interventions focused on the individual may need to yield to those that improve the economic and social circumstances of communities more generally. Other options may involve creating a "surrogate" community—for example, bringing together and sustaining a support group of poor single mothers through a local church—for populations in need that can support and sustain individuals.

The urgency to consider the effects of market changes and managed care is dawning on communities as well (Steinberg and Baxter, 1998). A review of how twelve local areas are responding to health care market forces revealed great concern among these communities that they were "losing control" of their provider resources. Respondents voiced common concerns that the primary missions that were valued by the community would be overtaken by financial and market pressures to cut costs and maximize profit. Communities could counter this concern if they could form or maintain a common set of values, which in turn would allow them to hold managed care and their providers accountable for upholding and being consistent with those values. Lack of community cohesiveness left them more subject to control by external forces and more instability in health care.

Efforts such as the Healthy Cities and Healthy Communities programs, which are supported from a variety of sources, have focused on developing capacity through public-private coalitions at the local level. These programs cover not only health but extend into priority areas set by residents, businesses, and others. These priority areas significantly affect health and include housing, education, and economic disparities. They share a common purpose of raising the condition of the total community.

Finally, many of these recommendations share one common shortcoming: a need for more information to assess the effect of managed care on the inner city, its diverse residents, and its traditional providers of care. In identifying this need, we call for the creation of a national strategy that uses the policy areas and the significant expertise in the areas of managed care, urban health, and its related service organizations and professionals to monitor the transitional and long-term implications on quality and access to care in our nation's urban areas. Targeted areas for this strategy include tracking the effect of state policies on these communities, including changes in support for the safety net and expanded coverage of urban populations to determine whether needed services and health care access generally are available and used. It should create options for the role of the urban safety net as well as document what has not worked. The strategy should assess the effect of expansion and contraction of managed care organizations accepting Medicaid enrollees on inner-city communities. It should also document the impact on broader community services such as public health surveillance of diseases and high cost–low profit services such as emergency care.

Conclusion

Creating consistent and positive directions within managed care that lead to a more equitable health care system and better health for urban residents amid rapidly changing, and at times disorderly, circumstances represents the greatest challenge to those responsible for providing health care, setting policy, and overseeing service programs. Ultimately all of these actions come down to what is best for the health of individuals and their communities.

Two directions seem to be emerging regarding the role of managed care entities in the inner city. One is the managed care organization working to become a true community program, considering how support can best be organized to meet inner-city needs. In this scenario, managed care organizations tend to make a longer-term investment in the community. In the second scenario, the managed care organization functions largely as a fiscal intermediary—a banker, contract negotiator, marketer—often for only as long as a profit is realized. One key question concerns the extent to which those involved with managed care can translate their commitment into a broader vision of responsibility.

In all, managed care and affiliated organizations could be the missing piece of the universal access puzzle since they represent the entities that can coordinate care, monitor services and quality, instill accountability, control costs, and predict service needs—activities that in their entirety were not performed under fee-for-service. There may also be a reciprocal benefit in the interrelationships. In order to survive in urban areas, managed care organizations need to establish connections with traditional community providers, as well as establish commitment to the community—a sort of civic conscience. This does not necessarily mean that they have to be nonprofit. However, they do have to give something to the community. Developing a civic conscience requires focusing on more than just the premium. It requires focusing on the community itself. When the organization takes an interest in the community and does not appear to be invested in this area solely for premium payments, the inner-city population may be less wary of its intentions.

The opportunity for significant, positive change to be derived from managed care for those in our cities cannot be overstated: the ability to mainstream individuals who have been permanently on the periphery of the health care system. But to make sustainable progress, managed care plans and providers will need to transform the frequently anecdotal stories of success and attention to the inner city into documented strategies across systems and communities. At the same time, evaluation of effectiveness to fill a void in information will grow in importance. Two secondary but nonetheless very important opportunities are often overlooked: to mainstream a provider system that has been on the periphery as well and to bring managed health care organizations and other providers into the mainstream of caring for the community as a whole. How to turn these opportunities into reality is the challenge confronting those committed to working toward the highest-quality health care system.

Appendix A:
The U.S. Teaching Hospital Survey on Managed Care in Urban Areas

ID Information

Hospital Name: _____

Address: _____

AHA ID#: _____

Name of person filling out form/contact person _____

Title: _____

Phone: _____

Fax: _____

E-mail: _____

Indicate dates of most recently closed fiscal year ___/___/___ — ___/___/___

Part I

A. General Hospital Characteristics

1. With which components of an integrated system does your hospital currently own or contract? Answer each line. (See Table A.1.)

2. Has your hospital undergone a change in governance in the last five years?

   Yes_____   No_____

If yes, what was your hospital's previous form of governance?

   a. Direct operation from state or local government

   b. Separate board within a government entity

   c. Hospital authority

   d. Hospital district

   e. Public benefit hospital corporation

Table A.1.
Components of an Integrated Delivery System

	Own	Contract for service	In the next two years, plan to create or buy	Don't know
a. Ambulatory surgery				
b. Community health centers				
c. Dental care				
d. Dialysis				
e. Health maintenance organization				
f. Home health care				
g. Hospice care				
h. Inpatient care				
i. Inpatient mental health care				
j. Inpatient substance abuse treatment				
k. Long-term-care nursing home beds				
l. Outpatient mental health care				
m. Outpatient pharmacies				
n. Outpatient substance abuse treatment				
o. Physician practices located in the community				
p. Primary care, located at hospital				
q. Public health clinics				
r. Rehabilitation beds				
s. Specialty outpatient care				
t. Subacute care				
u. Vision care				

f. Nonprofit hospital corporation

g. For-profit hospital corporation

h. Other/Specify _____

i. Don't know

3. In the next two years, do you believe you will have to undergo
major structural changes to compete?

Yes _____   No _____   Unable to judge _____

If so, please specify.

_____

_____

_____

4. How does your hospital provide the following services? Answer each line.
(See Table A.2.)

5. Does your hospital perform case management for the following?
Answer each line. (See Table A.3.)
(Case management is defined as an organized program that coordinates
individual patient care throughout the entire spectrum of services with
the goal of providing quality care in the most effective manner.)

B: Physician Practice

6. Please indicate the affiliation arrangements of your physician staff.
Answer each line. (See Table A.4.)

7. What is the ratio of full-time active primary care staff to full-time active
specialty care staff in your hospital?

_____ / _____

number of primary   number of specialty
care staff   care staff

Table A.2.
Provision of Special Services

	Directly provide	Contract for service	Plan to provide	Do not provide	Don't know
a. Assistance in obtaining housing					
b. Child care for patients					
c. Counseling for domestic and/or sexual abuse					
d. Cultural sensitivity training for staff					
e. Homeless assistance outreach workers					
f. Interpreter/translator services					
g. Other services					
h. Public health functions					
i. Transportation services					
j. Violence prevention program					
k. WIC office					

Table A.3.
Case Management

	Directly provide	Contract with	Plan to provide	Do not provide	Don't know
a. Complex medical cases					
b. Nonurgent use of the emergency department					
c. Repeat users of the emergency department					
d. Patients with HIV/AIDS					
e. Patients with mental illness					
f. Pediatric patients with chronic illnesses					
g. Substance abuse patients					
h. For other medical conditions? Please specify below:					

Table A.4.
Physician Staff

	Directly provide	Contract with	Plan to provide	Do not provide	Don't know
a. Foundation					
b. Group practice without walls					
c. Independent practice association					
d. Management service organization					
e. Physician-hospital organization					
f. Salaried staff					
g. Other					

Part II: Managed Care Characteristics
of the Service Area and Hospital

8. Circle the letter that best describes the managed care market
   classification of your service area. We are using the University
   HealthSystem Consortium classifications.

   a. Unstructured system: Primarily fee-for-service with little managed
      care contracting—less than 10 percent managed care in the market.
      Discounting for hospitals is generally in the 5–10 percent range, and
      there is little to no physician integration.

   b. Loose Framework: Managed care in the form of HMOs and PPOs
      becoming increasingly acceptable; estimated 10–24 percent managed
      care in the market. Discounting for hospitals typically falls in the
      15–25 percent range, and IPAs develop for PPO contracting.
      Utilization management efforts by payers lead to reduced hospital
      use rates and occupancy.

   c. Consolidation: HMO concentration reaches 25–49 percent in the
      market. Utilization risk shifts to capitated payment arrangements.
      HMOs mature and consolidate, physician "groups" develop and grow,
      and the competitive focus is on cost per covered life.

   d. Managed Competition: HMOs and PPOs dominate the market—
      managed care exceeds 50 percent in the market. Integrated delivery
      networks accept and manage fully capitated contracts, long-term
      services management contracts to Group Practices Without Walls are
      prevalent, and there is employment or capitation of group practices.

   e. Unable to judge.

9. In the year 2000, estimate under which managed care market classification
   you believe your service area will fall. (Same definitions as found in
   question 8.)

   a. Unstructured

   b. Loose framework

   c. Consolidation

   d. Managed competition

   e. Unable to judge

10. How does your hospital participate in managed care? Answer each line.
    a. Own a managed care plan
    b. Partner in a managed care plan
    c. Contract with managed care plans to provide services on a capitated basis
    d. Contract with managed care plans to provide services on a noncapitated basis
    e. Do not participate in any managed care arrangements
    f. Other relationships; specify _____
    g. Do not know

11. In the past two years, indicate the extent to which the following have been impediments for increasing managed care contracting at your hospital. Please rank in order of importance, with "1" being the most significant factor and "13" being the least significant factor.

Impediments	*Ranking*
a. Dominance of specialty care	
b. High cost of services	
c. Hospital location	
d. Inaccessible primary care sites	
e. Inadequate amenities	
f. Inadequate capital	
g. Inadequate delivery system integration	
h. Inadequate information systems	
i. Inadequate managed care expertise by medical staff	
j. Inadequate managed care expertise by nonphysician staff	
k. Inadequate primary care capacity	
l. Statutory or regulatory regulations	
m. No single contracting entity for hospital and physician services	

Part III: Hospital Financial Characteristics

12. Please estimate the percentage of the patient revenues derived from all types of managed care contracts in fiscal year 1996. Check most appropriate.
    a. Less than 5 percent
    b. 6–10 percent
    c. 11–20 percent
    d. 21–30 percent
    e. 31–50 percent
    f. 51–75 percent
    g. 76–100 percent

(If possible, please provide the amount of corresponding charged-based revenues for managed care contracts for FY 1996: $ _____)

13. Please estimate the percentage of patient charges represented by self-pay/charity/uninsured patients in fiscal year 1996. Check most appropriate.
    a. Less than 5 percent
    b. 6–10 percent
    c. 11–20 percent
    d. 21–30 percent
    e. 31–50 percent
    f. 51–75 percent
    g. 76–100 percent

(If possible, please provide the amount of corresponding charged-based revenues for self/charity/uninsured contracts for FY 1996: $ _____)

14. By the year 2000 what percentage of your hospital's revenue do you estimate will be derived from managed care?
    a. Less than 5 percent
    b. 6–10 percent
    c. 11–20 percent
    d. 21–30 percent
    e. 31–50 percent

f. 51–75 percent

g. 76–100 percent

h. Unable to judge

(If possible, please provide the amount of corresponding charged-based gross revenues for managed care contracts for FY 1996: $ _____)

15. If you received any capitated payments directly from payers, did the payments have:

Adjustments to Capitated Payments	Capitated payments from Medicare	Capitated payments from Medicaid	Capitated payments from HMO plans
a. Special allowance or adjustments for high-risk patients?			
b. Special allowance or adjustments for direct medical education?			
c. Special allowance or adjustments for indirect medical education?			
d. Special allowance or adjustments for DSH?			
e. Other adjustments? Please describe:			

Part IV: How Managed Care Affects Services, Delivery, and Access

16. In your opinion, during the past two years, please indicate the status of the following in your service area. (See Table A.5.)

17. In the next two years, what changes do you foresee for your hospital? Answer each line. (See Table A.6.)

18. In your opinion, at your hospital, how has managed care affected the utilization of services for each of the categories in Table A.7?

Part V: Graduate Medical Education

19. Please indicate, for each of the specialty areas that follow, whether your hospital has changed the number of positions and/or is anticipating a change in the next five years.

    1 = increase; 2 = decrease; 3 = no change/not applicable

Specialties	Area	During 1997	Within the next five years
Anesthesiology			
Emergency Medicine			
Family Practice			
Internal Medicine			
Medicine Subspecialties			
Obstetrics and Gynecology			
Pathology			
Pediatrics			
Pediatric Subspecialties			
Psychiatry			
Radiology			
Surgery			
Surgical Subspecialties			
Other (please specify):			

Table A.5. Changes in Percentage of Uninsured	Significantly increased	Increased	No change	Decrease	Significantly decreased
a. The percentage of uninsured patients that use your hospital					
b. The percentage of other community providers treating "high-risk" patients					
c. The available funds for the financing of uninsured patients					

Table A.6. Organizational Changes Anticipated in the Next Two Years	Will happen	Likely to happen	Unlikely to happen	Will not happen	Unable to judge
a. Close beds					
b. Develop community-based satellite facilities					
c. Downsize medical staff					
d. Downsize nonphysician staff					
e. Downsize residency programs					
f. Improve systems and infrastructure for managing patient care					
g. Increase primary care capacity					
h. Market specialty networks					
i. New capital projects					

Table A.7. Utilization Changes

	Increased	Hasn't changed	Decreased	Don't know
a. Adults with chronic conditions				
b. Beneficiaries with commercial insurance				
c. Children with chronic conditions				
d. Individuals with chronic mental illness				
e. Medicare recipients				
f. Medicaid recipients				
g. Patients who need primary care				
h. Patients who need specialty care				
i. The uninsured				

20. For programs that have decreased or you are contemplating decreasing the number of residency positions, please indicate the importance of the factors found in Table A.8.

21. How do the factors listed in Table A.9. affect your hospital's policy to increase or decrease resident positions? (Note: We recognize that some of your responses may be related to specific resident categories, such as primary care.)

Part VI: Emergency Department

For many emergency departments (EDs) authorization requirements and inappropriate patient transfers—that is, patients transferred from other hospitals based on insurance status or inability to pay (otherwise known as "patient dumping")—are major concerns. Please respond to the following related questions.

22. Please estimate trends in inappropriate patient transfers since January 1, 1996.
    a. Significant, major increase
    b. Small increase
    c. No change
    d. Small decrease
    e. Significant, major decrease

23. If your ED has witnessed a change since January 1, 1996, to what extent do you attribute that change to the influence of managed care?
    a. The major reason
    b. A minor reason
    c. Not a factor
    d. Do not know

24. To what extent do you estimate that pre- and postauthorization requirements imposed by managed care programs in which you do not participate create significant problems for your emergency department in treating enrollees?
    a. Have created major financial problems
    b. Have created moderate financial problems
    c. Have created limited financial problems
    d. Have created few or no problems

Table A.8.
Factors Affecting Residency Programs

Factors Affecting Residency Programs	Critical and primary	Very important	Important	Limited importance	Not a factor
a. Collaboration with other centers or consortia					
b. Difficulty in sustaining program quality					
c. Difficulty in filling positions with qualified applicants					
d. Desire to reduce the number of international medical graduates					
e. Shift time or positions to ambulatory care settings					
f. Difficulty of program graduates to find a job					
g. Decreased need for specialists					
h. Reduced need for house staff coverage for inpatients					
i. Decrease number and mix of patients available for teaching programs					
j. Pressure to reduce costs					
k. Possible changes in DME and IME financing					
l. Unwillingness of private payers to support GME costs					
m. Loss of Medicare or Medicaid GME payments as patients shifted into managed care					
n. Teaching physician physical presence and documentation requirements					
o. Need to compete with nonteaching hospitals					
p. Federal, state, or local reduction incentive or transition payment programs to encourage position reductions					
q. Other (please specify):					

Table A.9. Factors Affecting Recruitment	Very strong incentive to increase	Incentive to increase	Not a factor	Incentive to decrease	Very strong incentive to decrease
a. Ability to recruit qualified applicants					
b. Collaboration with other centers or consortia					
c. Cost effectiveness of housestaff compared to other providers					
d. Financial benefits of current GME financing					
e. Increased need for ambulatory experience for residents					
f. Increased need for primary care physicians					
g. Need for housestaff coverage for patient care needs					
h. Need to compete with non-teaching hospitals					
i. Potential ____ or Enacted ____ (please check one or both) federal, state, or local actions to encourage position reductions					
j. Program quality					
k. Role of residents in covering services on nights, weekends					
l. Uncertainty about the timing of changes in DME and IME financing					

25. For 1996, please estimate the amount of uncollected emergency department charges due to authorization denials of emergency department care by managed care companies. $ _____

26. Please estimate the total percent of emergency department charges represented by these denials. _____ percent

PLEASE RETURN THIS SURVEY TO:
[. . .]

Definition List

Capitation A set amount of money received or paid out; based on membership rather than on services delivered and usually is expressed in units of per member per month. The amount is fixed, assuming a certain level of utilization and cost per unit of service, thus shifting the risk of higher-than-expected utilization to the provider. It may be varied by such factors as age and sex of the enrolled member.

Charity care Health services that were never expected to result in cash inflow. Charity care results from a provider's policy to provide health care services free of charge to individuals who meet certain financial criteria.

Equity model Allows established practitioners to become shareholders in a professional corporation in exchange for tangible and intangible assets of their existing practices.

Foundation A corporation, organized as either a hospital affiliate or a subsidiary, that purchases both the tangible and intangible assets of one or more medical group practices. Physicians remain in a separate corporate entity but sign a professional services agreement with the foundation.

GPWW (Group Practice Without Walls) Hospital sponsors the formation of, or provides capital to physicians to establish, a "quasi" group to share administrative expenses while remaining independent practitioners.

HMO (Health Maintenance Organization) A prepaid organization that provides health care to voluntary enrolled members in return for a preset amount of money on a per member per month basis. Also includes the following elements: a health plan that places at least some of its providers at risk for medical expenses, and a health plan that utilizes primary care physicians as gatekeepers.

Integrated salary model Physicians are salaried by the hospital or another entity of a health system to provide medical services for primary care and specialty care.

IPA (Independent Practice Association) An organization that has a contract with a managed care plan to deliver services in return for a single capitation rate. The IPA in turn contracts with individual providers to provide services, on a capitation basis or a fee-for-service basis.

Managed care A system of health care delivery where the provision of an agreed-on set of health care services is coordinated by an entity or person (a health plan, includes PPOs, or primary care case manager) obligated by contract or other agreement to be responsible for the care provided (or not provided) to an individual.

MSO (Management Services Organization) Organization that provides administrative services to health care providers. Commonly created by hospitals to assist their affiliated physicians in the administrative aspects of their practices.

Own Individual ownership of services, agencies, and centers or belonging to a hospital network that owns these entities.

PHO (Physician-Hospital Organization) Legal (or perhaps informal) organizations that bond hospitals and the attending medical staff. Frequently develop for the purpose of contracting with managed care plans.

PPO (Preferred Provider Organization) A plan that contracts with independent providers at a discount for services. The panel is limited in size and usually has some type of utilization review system associated with it. It may be either risk bearing or nonrisk bearing.

Appendix B: Survey Data

Survey data were collected from a nonprobability sample of public and teaching hospitals based on two hospital association memberships: the National Association of Public Hospitals and Health Systems (NAPH) and the Council of Teaching Hospitals (COTH).

Data were collected to determine (1) hospitals' adaptation to managed care and (2) the impact of managed care. Several analytical procedures were conducted. To determine adaptation to managed care, information was collected on hospital characteristics and graduate medical education. To examine effects of managed care, information was collected on managed care characteristics and impact. Selected bivariate analyses were conducted to measure strength of associations. Hospital ownership or structure is used as an independent variable in these analyses because, anecdotally, public hospitals are seen as lagging behind in adjusting to market dynamics. Hospital ownership was determined using the American Hospital Association's 1996 *Annual Survey of Hospitals* data file. Based on the code for type of hospital authority, hospital ownership was dichotomized into public and private hospitals. *Public hospitals* are hospitals operated by state, county, city, or hospital authority. *Private hospitals* are hospitals operated by churches, other nonprofits, individuals, partnerships, or corporations. Most of the bivariate results yielded by these analyses were not conclusive, confirming the preliminary and baseline nature of data. However, a few of the tests proved to be significant using the chi-square test of association. Data suggest that the structural effects of managed care may still be nascent.

Five cross-tabulations are presented: market classification by region, hospital ownership by noncapitated managed care contracts, percentage of patient revenues derived from managed care contracts, percentage of patient charges represented by self-pay, and physician practices located in community. Except for market classification by region, all the other distributions were significant.

Questionnaires of the U.S. Teaching Hospital Survey on Managed Care in Urban Areas (see Appendix A) were mailed to the hospital CEO with detailed instructions on completing the survey.

Hospitals were provided with a list of managed care definitions. Returned questionnaires were checked for consistency and completeness, and reliability checks were used to ensure consistency. Analyses were conducted using SPSS for Windows version 6.1.

Results

Overall, 330 urban-based hospitals were surveyed, with 117 responding, for a response rate of approximately 40 percent. Responding hospitals have an average bed size of 500 (standard deviation, 262) and are regionally representative of the sample. Thirty-eight hospitals responded from the Northeast and 22 hospitals from the North-Central; there were 33 and 24 responding hospitals or urban-based hospitals from the South and West, respectively. Table B.1 presents the regional distribution of public and private hospitals responding to the survey. Almost the same number of public and private hospitals responded to the survey.

Table B.1. Distribution of Respondents
by Region and Ownership

	Northeast	North-Central	South	West	Total Responding
Public	32.4% (12)	36.4 % (8)	57.6 % (19)	83.3 % (20)	59
Private	67.6% (26)	63.6 % (14)	42.4% (14)	16.7% (4)	58

Hospital Characteristics

Information on hospital characteristics include components of integrated delivery systems of hospitals, assistance services, case management procedures, and changes in status of selected service areas in the past two years.

Integrated Delivery Systems. Table B.2 presents information on nineteen aspects of an integrated system operated by urban-based hospitals. Data show that the majority of responding urban-based hospitals (range, 59 percent to 93 percent) own the components of an integrated health delivery system. Responding hospitals have a variety of arrangements for providing ambulatory care:

- Eighty-six percent reported owning or contracting with clinics.
- Eighty-two percent owned or contracted with physicians who practice in the community.
- Ninety-eight owned or contracted for primary care in the hospital.
- Eighty-eight owned or contracted for public health services. Questions were not asked about specific service volumes.
- The majority of urban-based hospitals owned or contracted with HMOs (85 percent) and nursing homes (80 percent). Few responding urban-based hospitals plan to create or buy these services.

Physician Practices Located in Community by Ownership. Location of physician practices in the community is one of key characteristics of ready adaptation to managed care. To determine how the traditional safety net providers, particularly public hospitals, are adjusting to managed care, we compared them to private hospitals. Figure B.1 shows that:

- Proportionately more private hospitals, 84 percent (42 of 50), own physician practices in the community, compared with 51 percent (20 of 39) of public hospitals.

Table B.2. Components of an Integrated Delivery Systems
Provided by AHCS

	Own	Contract for Service	Plan to Create/Buy	Own and Contract	Total Responding
Community health centers	70.0% (61)	16.0% (14)	9.2% (8)	3.4% (3)	86
Dental care	76.3% (74)	17.5% (17)	3.1% (3)	2.1% (2)	96
Dialysis	67.0% (69)	29.1% (30)	1.0% (1)	2.9% (3)	103
HMO	44.0% (37)	40.5% (34)	10.7% (9)	4.8% (4)	84
Home health care	58.5% (62)	31.1% (33)	7.5% (8)	0.9% (1)	104
Hospice care	40.7% (37)	51.6% (47)	6.6% (6)	1.1% (1)	91
Inpatient mental health	87.7% (93)	10.4% (11)	0.9% (1)	0.9% (1)	106
Inpatient substance abuse	70.2% (59)	25.0% (21)	3.6% (3)	1.2% (1)	84
Long-term-care nursing home beds	44.3% (35)	35.4% (28)	17.7% (14)	2.5% (2)	79
Outpatient mental health	81.6% (80)	15.3% (15)	2.0% (2)	1.0% (1)	98
Outpatient pharmacies	82.8% (82)	7.1% (7)	8.1% (8)	2.0% (2)	99
Outpatient substance abuse	69.3% (61)	20.5% (18)	9.1% (8)	1.1% (1)	88
Physician practices in community	66.3% (63)	15.8% (15)	12.6% (12)	4.2% (4)	94
Primary care in hospital	92.7% (101)	5.5% (6)		0.9% (1)	108
Public health clinics	61.5% (40)	26.2% (17)	12.3% (8)		65
Rehabilitation beds	78.5% (73)	15.1% (14)	5.4% (5)	1.1% (1)	93
Specialty outpatient care	90.7% (97)	6.5% (7)	1.9% (2)	0.9% (1)	107
Subacute care	59.8% (52)	17.2% (15)	20.7% (18)	2.3% (2)	87
Vision care	72.4% (63)	20.7% (18)	2.3% (2)	4.6% (4)	87

- Proportionately more public hospitals contract for physician service, 28 percent (11 of 39), compared with 8 percent (4 of 50) of private hospitals.

- Proportionately more public hospitals plan to create or buy these practices, 21 percent (8 of 39), than private hospitals, 8 percent (4 of 50). These distributions are significant.

Responding urban-based hospitals have a ratio of three specialists to one primary care physician.

Assistance Services. Beyond having integrated clinical services, an integrated delivery system that serves inner-city patients needs to offer assistance services. The surveyed hospitals offer or

Figure B.1. How AHCs Contract for Physician Services

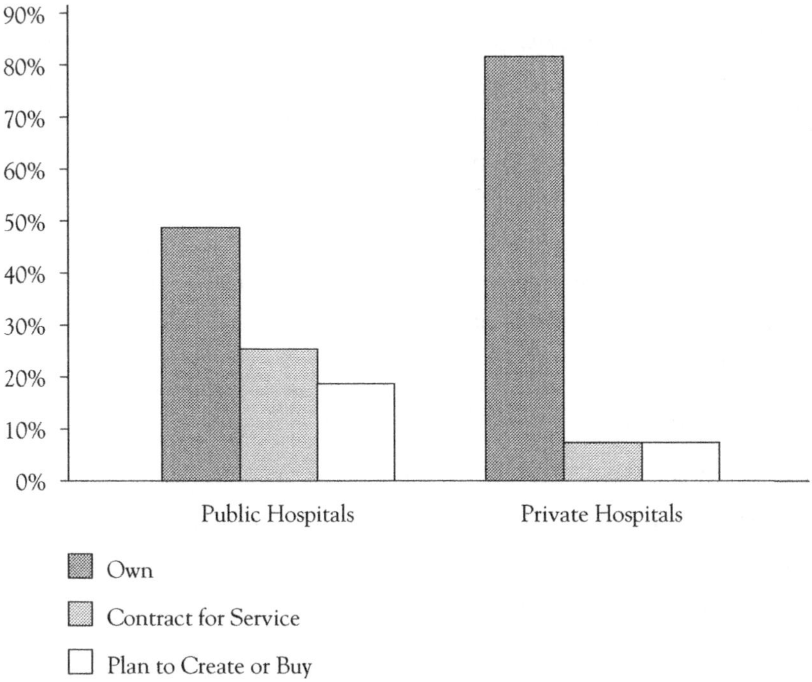

Note: $N = 89$, $p < 0.01$, $X^2 = 11$, $DF = 2$.

contract for a variety of assistance services that supplement clinical services (see Table B.3):

- Most responding hospitals provide counseling for domestic violence (77 percent).
- Most responding hospitals provide cultural sensitivity training for staff (87 percent) and interpreter/translator services (68 percent).
- The majority of hospitals provide public health services (64 percent) and violence prevention programs (62 percent).
- The majority of responding urban-based hospitals directly provided or contracted for transportation (74 percent) and WIC services (66 percent).
- The majority of responding hospitals do not provide assistance in obtaining housing for patients (52 percent), child care (76 percent), or homeless assistance outreach (55 percent).

Case Management. Case management is defined as an organized program that coordinates individual patient care throughout the entire spectrum of services with the goal of providing quality care in the most effective manner. It is critical for managing utilization of health services. The survey documents that more than half of the hospitals offered some type of case management services. Data on case management procedures are presented in Table B.4. Overall the vast majority of hospitals directly provided case management for:

- Complex medical cases (74 percent)
- Patients with HIV/AIDS (73 percent)
- Nonurgent use of the emergency room (54 percent)
- Patients with mental illness (59 percent)
- Pediatric patients with chronic illness (56 percent)

However, a sizable proportion of respondents do not provide case management for:

Table B.3. Types of Assistance Services Provided by AHCs

	Directly Provide	Contract Service	Plan to Provide	Don't Provide	Total Responding
Assistance in obtaining housing	35.2% (38)	9.3% (10)		51.9% (56)	104
Child care for patients	11.5% (12)	7.7% (8)	4.8% (5)	76.0% (79)	104
Counseling for domestic violence	76.8% (86)	8.0% (9)	1.8% (2)	9.8% (11)	108
Cultural sensitivity training for staff	87.0% (100)	2.6% (3)	6.1% (7)	2.6% (3)	113
Homeless assistance outreach	30.8% (32)	11.5% (12)	2.9% (3)	54.8% (57)	104
Interpreter/translator services	68.1% (77)	9.7% (11)	0.9% (1)	2.7% (3)	92
Public health functions	63.5% (61)	9.4% (9)	1.0% (1)	24.0% (23)	94
Transportation services	40.2% (45)	33.9% (38)	2.7% (3)	15.2% (17)	103
Violence prevention programs	61.5% (64)	5.8% (6)	7.7% (8)	24.0% (25)	103
WIC office	45.2% (47)	21.2% (22)	1.9% (2)	30.8% (32)	103

- Substance abuse patients (25 percent)
- Nonurgent use of the emergency room (24 percent)
- Repeat users of the emergency room (22 percent)

Status of Uninsured. The survey showed that in the past two years:

- A slight majority of urban-based hospitals (51 percent) experienced increases in the percentage of uninsured patients.
- A substantial proportion of respondents reported no change (45 percent).
- Nevertheless, 59 percent reported a decrease in available funds for financing uninsured patients.

These status changes are reported in Table B.5.

Graduate Medical Education

Graduate medical education data are represented by factors affecting residency positions and changes in number of positions in specialty areas.

Factors Affecting Residency. Table B.6 provides information on the factors that affect residency programs:

- Clearly, the key factor among the twelve listed that influences increases in residency programs is increased need for primary care physicians, with 70 percent of responding urban-based hospitals indicating this.
- Of the factors listed as affecting residency positions, the majority of responding urban-based hospitals indicated that two were nonfactors: the need to compete with nonteaching hospitals (55 percent) and the role or residents in covering services (52 percent).

Table B.4. Case Management Services Provided by AHCs

	Directly Provide	Contract with	Plan to Provide	Don't Provide	Provide and Contract	Total Responding
Complex medical cases	73.5% (83)	1.8% (2)	11.5% (13)	8.8% (10)	1.8% (2)	110
Nonurgent use of the ER	53.6% (59)	2.7% (3)	18.2% (20)	23.6% (26)	1.8% (2)	110
Repeat users of the ER	48.6% (52)	3.7% (4)	23.4% (25)	21.5% (23)	1.9% (2)	106
Patients with HIV/AIDS	72.7% (80)	2.7% (3)	6.4% (7)	13.6% (15)	4.5% (5)	110
Patients with mental illness	59.4% (63)	8.5% (9)	7.5% (8)	17.9% (19)	6.6% (7)	106
Pediatric patients with chronic illness	56.2% (59)	7.6% (8)	9.5% (10)	20.0% (21)	4.8% (5)	103
Substance abuse patients	48.5% (49)	11.9% (12)	10.9% (11)	24.8% (25)	4.0% (4)	101
For other medical conditions	79.5% (35)		4.5% (2)	9.1% (4)	6.8% (3)	44

Table B.5. Changes in Percentage of Uninsured Using AHCs

	Increased	No Change	Decreased	Total Responding
Percentage of uninsured patients who use hospital	50.9% (57)	44.6% (50)	4.5% (5)	112
Available funds for financing uninsured patients	9.8% (11)	31.0% (35)59	.3% (67)	113

Table B.6. Factors Affecting Number of Residency Positions

	Incentive to Increase	Not a Factor	Incentive to Decrease	Total Responding
Ability to recruit qualified applicants	29.4% (30)	35.3% (36)	35.3% (36)	102
Collaboration with other centers	20.0% (20)	47.0% (47)	32.0% (32)	100
Cost-effectiveness of house staff	45.5% (45)	38.4% (38)	16.2% (16)	99
Financial benefits of current GME financing	39.2% (40)	27.5% (28)	31.4% (32)	102
Increased need for ambulatory experience	37.0% (37)	46.0% (46)	17.0% (17)	100
Increased need for a primary care physician	70.0% (70)	25.0% (25)	5.0% (5)	100
Need for house staff coverage for patient care	43.0% (43)	49.0% (49)	8.0% (8)	100
Need to compete with nonteaching hospitals	9.9% (10)	55.4% (56)	33.6% (34)	101
Federal or state actions to encourage reductions	11.20% (11)	32.7% (32)	56.2% (55)	98
Program quality	30.9% (30)	43.3% (42)	23.7% (23)	97
Role of residents in covering services	45.6% (46)	51.5% (52)	2.0% (2)	101
Uncertainty about the timing of change	6.0% (6)	39.0% (39)	55.0% (55)	100

- Federal or state actions to encourage reductions and uncertainty about timing of change in the market are two factors that lead to reductions in residency positions according to a majority of respondents (56 percent and 55 percent, respectively).
- Distribution of responses to the other factors was not concentrated. For instance, whereas 46 percent of respondents indicated that cost-effectiveness of house staff was an incentive to increase residency positions, a considerable percentage, 38 percent, did not regard this as a factor. Whereas 47 percent of respondents judged collaboration with other centers to be a nonfactor, 32 percent regarded this factor as influencing reductions in positions. The same pattern of diffusion in responses is palpable for the following factors: ability to recruit qualified applicants, financial benefits of current GME financing, increased need for ambulatory experience, need for house staff coverage for patient care, and program quality.

Changes in Number of Positions in Specialty.   From Table B.7 we can see that:

- Overall, there have not been changes in the number of positions in thirteen key specialty areas in the majority of responding hospitals (range, 56 percent to 82 percent).
- In very few cases are training programs going to increase. However, a considerable percentage of hospitals, 31 percent, expect to increase family medicine.

Managed Care Participation and Impact

To illustrate the extent of managed care penetration and impact, data are presented on market classification, how urban-based hospitals participate in managed care, impediments for increasing managed care, affiliation agreements with physician staff and anticipated structural changes in the next two years, and how managed care has affected utilization and revenues.

Table B.7. Changes in Number of Residency Positions in the Next Five Years

	Incentive to Increase	Not a Factor	Incentive to Decrease	Total Responding
Anesthesiology	6.1% (6)	38.4% (38)	55.6% (55)	99
Emergency medicine	14.9% (14)	3.2% (3)	81.9% (77)	94
Family medicine	30.9% (30)	3.1% (3)	66.0% (64)	97
Internal medicine	14.2% (15)	12.3% (13)	73.6% (78)	106
Medicine subspecialties	1.0% (1)	34.3% (34)	64.6% (64)	99
Obstetrics and gynecology	10.7% (11)	12.6% (13)	76.7% (79)	103
Pathology	4.0% (4)	29.0% (29)	67.0% (67)	100
Pediatrics	13.1% (13)	13.1% (13)	73.7% (73)	99
Pediatric subspecialty	9.0% (8)	13.5% (12)	77.5% (69)	89
Psychiatry	6.3% (6)	21.9% (21)	71.9% (69)	96
Radiology	10.2% (10)	18.4% (18)	71.4% (70)	98
Surgery	8.7% (9)	17.5% (18)	73.8% (76)	103
Surgery subspecialties	5.4% (5)	15.1% (14)	79.6% (74)	93

Managed Care Market Classification. From Table B.8 we can see that full-fledged managed competition has not taken place in the health care market as yet (the market classification is based on a model developed by the University Health Consortium, or UHC):

- A slight majority of responding hospitals report operating in a loose or unstructured market framework (44 percent)— one with less than 10 percent to 24 percent managed care in the market.

- Considerable proportions of respondents operate in a consolidated market (40 percent), with an HMO concentration of 25 percent to 49 percent in the market.

- Only 14 percent of respondents reportedly operate in a market dominated by HMOs and PPOs (50 percent or more concentration in the market).

Table B.8. Changes in Managed Care Market Classification,
1996–2000

	Loose Framework	Consolidation	Managed Competition	Unable to Judge	Total Responding
Market classification in 1996	43.5% (50)	40.0% (46)	13.9% (16)	2.6% (3)	115
Market classification in year 2000	4.3% (5)	40.5% (47)	51.7% (60)	3.4% (4)	116

- By the year 2000, 52 percent of responding urban-based hospitals believed they would be operating in a managed competition market, and 41 percent believed they would be operating in a consolidated market.

Managed Care Market by Region. When hospitals are considered regionally, the survey showed:

- Clearly managed care has seen the most growth in the West. Approximately 52 percent (11 of 21) of urban-based hospitals in the West operate in a managed competition market compared with 6 percent (2 of 33) in the South, 5 percent (1 of 37) in the Northeast, and 5 percent (2 of 21) in the North-Central (see Figure B.2).

- Most hospitals in the Northeast operate in a consolidated market (54 percent, or 20 of 37).

- Indeed, a considerable proportion of hospitals in the West (38 percent, or 8 of 21) also operates in a consolidated market.

- The majority of hospitals in the North-Central and the South operate in an unstructured or loose framework: 62 percent (13 of 21) and 61 percent (20 of 33), respectively.

- Forty-one percent (41 percent, or 15 of 37) of hospitals in the Northeast report operating in a loose framework.

Figure B.2. Managed Care Market Classification
by Region

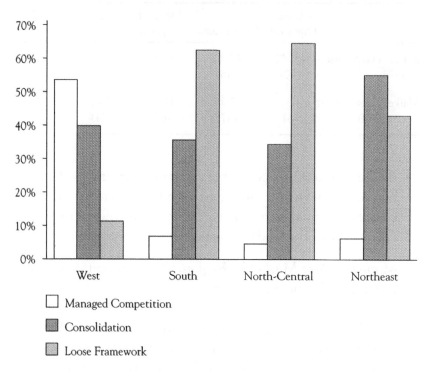

Participation in Managed Care. Table B.9 presents data on how urban-based hospitals participate in managed care:

- Approximately 70 percent responding to the survey do not own managed care plans.
- Approximately 59 percent are not partners in plans either.
- A majority of responding hospitals contract with a managed care organizations only on a capitated basis (72 percent).
- Eighty-four percent contract on a noncapitated basis.
- Ninety-two percent of respondents are engaged in other relationships involving managed care (only one reporting hospital does not participate in any plan).

Table B.9. How AHCs Participate in Managed Care

	Yes	No	Total Responding
Own a managed care plan	31.0% (36)	69.0% (80)	116
Partner in a managed care plan	42.2% (49)	57.8% (67)	116
Contract with managed care plans on a capitated basis	71.6% (83)	28.4% (33)	116
Contract with managed care plans on a noncapitated basis	83.6% (97)	16.4% (19)	116
Do not participate in any managed care arrangement	0.9% (1)	99.1%) (115	116
Other relationships	7.8% (9)	92.2% (107)	116

Currently all hospitals are challenged by receiving different types of reimbursement that provide incentives to an organization to behave in different ways. To maximize fee-for-service revenues, institutions may want to treat high-risk patients and provide as many services as are medically appropriate.

On the other hand, if hospitals are compensated as managed care plans on a capitated basis, their incentive is to care for low-risk patients and provide the fewest number of services that are medically appropriate. Currently when reimbursement is changing from one that is predominantly fee-for-service to one that is managed care, providers are challenged to develop strategic approaches to maximize both fee-for-service and managed care reimbursement.

Contract with Managed Care by Ownership. To determine whether strategies for contracting to maximize reimbursement vary by hospital structure, we compared public with private hospitals. Figure B.3 depicts the distribution of public and private hospitals by noncapitated managed care service contracts.

**Figure B.3 Percentage of Noncapitated Managed Care Contracts,
by Hospital Ownership**

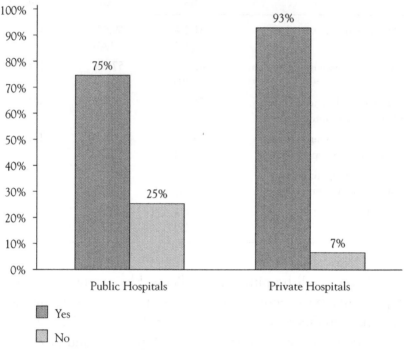

Note: N = 115, *p* < 0.01, X^2 = 7, DF = 1.

- There are proportionately more private hospitals contracting
  on a noncapitated basis, 93 percent (52 of 56), compared with
  75 percent (44 of 59) of public hospitals. This distribution is
  significant.

This distribution may reflect managed care organizations' seeking out private hospitals and private hospitals' having greater desire
and flexibility to contract.

To capture managed care revenues, teaching and public hospitals will need to make strategic and organizational changes. The
survey inquired as to what types of changes would be necessary and
what impediments the institutions face.

Impediments for Increasing Managed Care. When compared to other factors thwarting the expansion of managed care:

- High cost of services was the factor that a considerable proportion of responding urban-based hospitals (40 percent) judged to be an impediment, followed by:
- Dominance of specialty care (23 percent) and
- Lack of single contracting entity for hospital (21 percent). Of note, however, is the fact that a sizable percentage of responding urban-based hospitals did not consider the lack of single contracting entity as an impediment.

These data are presented in Table B.10.

How Managed Care Affects Utilization. Of the nine areas of utilization, the majority of responding urban-based hospitals have experienced no change in the following six areas:

- Adults with chronic conditions (63 percent)
- Children with chronic conditions (62 percent)
- Individuals with chronic mental illness (50 percent)
- Medicare recipients (52 percent)
- Patients who need specialty care (53 percent)
- The uninsured (57 percent)

Of significance, however, is the fact that approximately 55 percent of respondents report that the number of beneficiaries with commercial insurance has decreased, 58 percent report that the number of patients needing primary care has increased, and 42 percent report that the number of Medicaid patients has decreased. Data are presented in Table B.11.

Anticipated Changes in Next Two Years. In the context of the growing influence of managed care in the health market, it is important to note the kinds of strategies that hospitals are using or

Table B.10. Impediments for Increasing Managed Care Contacts

	Most Important	Less Important	Total Responding
Dominance of specialty care	23.0% (23)	12.0% (12)	100
High cost of services	40.8% (42)	13.6% (14)	103
Hospital location	12.7% (12)	21.0% (20)	95
Inaccessible primary care sites	8.3% (8)	14.6% (14)	96
Inadequate amenities	8.3% (8)	15.4% (15)	97
Inadequate capital	7.3% (7)	17.7 % (17)	96
Inadequate delivery system integration	19.2% (19)	6.0% (6)	99
Inadequate information systems	19.2% (19)	3.0% (3)	99
Inadequate experience by physician staff	13.0% (13)	5.0% (5)	100
Inadequate experience by nonphysician staff	7.0% (7)	14.2% (14)	99
Inadequate primary care capacity	16.7% (16)	5.9% (6)	102
Statutory or regulatory	12.1% (12)	35.3% (35)	99
No single contracting entity for hospital	21.4% (21)	37.7% (37)	98

Table B.11. How Managed Care Has Affected Utilization
at AHCs

	Increased	Hasn't Changed	Decreased	Total Responding
Adults with chronic conditions	14.9% (14)	62.8% (59)	22.3% (21)	94
Beneficiaries with commercial insurance	7.7% (8)	37.5% (39)	54.8% (57)	104
Children with chronic conditions	15.2% (12)	62.0% (49)	22.8% (18)	79
Individuals with chronic mental illness	15.0% (12)	50.0% (40)	33.8% (27)	80
Medicare recipients	13.6% (14)	52.4% (54)	31.1% (32)	103
Medicaid recipients	22.3% (23)	34.0% (35)	41.7% (43)	103
Patients who need primary care	58.2% (57)	31.6% (31)	9.2% (9)	98
Patients who need specialty care	26.5% (26)	53.1% (52)	20.4% (20)	98
The uninsured	34.3% (34)	56.6% (56)	9.1% (9)	99

planning to undertake to compete. Table B.12 shows that in the next two years, most urban-based hospitals anticipate:

- A reduction of beds (61 percent)
- Downsizing nonphysician staff (71 percent)
- Downsizing residency programs (57 percent)

On the other hand, most responding urban-based hospitals anticipate:

- Developing community facilities (87 percent)
- Improving systems and infrastructure (100 percent)
- Increasing primary care capacity (94 percent)
- Marketing specialty networks (89 percent)

**Table B.12. Organization Changes Anticipated in the
Next Two Years to Respond to Managed Care**

	Will Happen/ Likely to Happen	Unlikely to Happen/ Will Not Happen	Total Responding
Close beds	60.5% (69)	32.4% (37)	106
Develop community-based satellite facilities	86.8% (98)	10.7% (12)	110
Downsize medical staff	34.2% (39)	56.2% (64)	103
Downsize nonphysician staff	71.1% (79)	21.6% (24)	103
Downsize residency programs	57.1% (64)	32.2% (36)	100
Improve systems and infrastructure	100.0% (104)		104
Increase primary care capacity	93.8% (107)	5.3% (6)	113
Market specialty networks	89.2% (99)	4.5% (5)	104
New capital projects	86.8% (99)	8.8% (10)	109

- Starting new capital projects (87 percent)
- Fifty-six percent of urban-based hospitals do not forecast a reduction in medical staff

Governance and Structural Changes. Hospitals that are implementing managed care often require capital and information systems. To raise capital and make quick decisions regarding information systems requires an institution to be organizationally nimble. This need to operate nimbly is documented by the following facts:

- Twenty-seven percent of the responding hospitals have changed their governance during the last five years.

- However, governance changes during the past five years still have not been sufficient for the surveyed hospitals; 56 percent of the surveyed hospitals still indicate a need for a major structural change in the next two years.
- Of the 64 hospitals that indicate a need for a major structural change, 27 percent (17) underwent a structural change as recently as five years ago.
- The hospitals that are most likely to undergo major structural changes are in loose or consolidated markets (44 percent [28] and 40 percent [25], respectively).

These data are presented in Table B.13.

Managed Care and Self-Pay Revenues. Table B.14 presents information on percentage of revenues derived from managed care and self-pay, charity, and uninsured:

- Only 5 percent (6) of responding urban-based hospitals derive the bulk of their revenues (51 percent to 75 percent) from managed care.
- Eight percent (9) state that most of their charges are related to self-pay, charity, or the uninsured.

Table B.13. Changes in Governance

	Yes	No	Unable to Judge	Total Responding
Governance changed in last five years	27.4% (32)	72.6% (85)		117
Major structural changes in next two years	56.1% (64)	32.5% (37)	11.4% (13)	114

Percentage of Patient Revenues from Managed Care by Ownership. Table B.15 shows estimates of patient revenues derived from managed care in 1996, as well as anticipated estimates in the year 2000 by hospital ownership or structure. In 1996 the distribution by ownership showed significance, whereas the estimates anticipated for 2000 were not significant by ownership. These data show that in 1996:

- A considerable proportion of public hospitals, 41 percent, derives less than 5 percent of patient revenues from managed care. Furthermore, 19 percent of public hospitals derive 6 to 10 percent of their revenues from managed care compared with only 5 percent of private hospitals.

- Overall, proportionately more private hospitals derive significant portions of their revenues from managed care: 73 percent of private hospitals acquire 20 to 75 percent of their revenues from managed care compared with 23 percent of public hospitals.

Percentage of Patient Charges Represented by Self-Pay by Ownership. Data in Table B.16 show that:

- Proportionately more public hospitals derive considerable portions of their patient charges from self-pay, charity, or uninsured: 57 percent of responding public hospitals acquire 20 to 75 percent of their revenues from self-pay, charity, or uninsured compared with 2 percent of private hospitals.

- The majority of responding private hospitals, 79 percent, derive up to 10 percent of their revenues from self-pay, charity, or uninsured.

Discussion

Findings from characteristics of respondents confirm the public health functions of public and teaching hospitals as well as the strides being made to improve services by these hospitals. The

Table B.14. Managed Care and Self-Pay Revenues

	Less Than 5%	6–10%	11–20%	21–30%	31–50%	51–75%	Total Responding
Number of patient revenues from managed care	20.9% (24)	12.2% (14)	19.1% (22)	27.8% (32)	14.8% (17)	5.2% (6)	115
Number of patients charges represented by self-pay[a]	25.0% (28)	23.2% (26)	22.3% (25)	10.7% (12)	10.7% (12)	8.0% (9)	112

[a] Includes charity and uninsured.

Table B.15. Percentage of Patient Revenues Derived from Managed Care Contracts

	Public Hospitals		Private Hospitals	
	Year 1996[a]	Year 2000	1996	Year 2000
Less than 5%	41% (24)	2% (1)	0%	0%
6–10%	19% (11)	9% (5)	5% (3)	0%
11–20%	17% (10)	20% (11)	21% (12)	4% (2)
21–30%	14% (8)	13% (7)	41% (23)	4% (2)
31–50%	7% (4)	36% (20)	23% (13)	65% (35)
51–75%	2% (1)	21% (12)	9% (5)	22% (12)
75–100%	0%	0%	0%	6% (3)

[a] $p < 0.01$, $X^2 = 43$, DF = 5 for 1996.

Table B.16. Percentage of Patient Self-Pay Revenues

	Public Hospitals	Private Hospitals
Less than 5%	5% (3)	46% (25)
6–10%	13% (7)	33% (18)
11–20%	25% (14)	20% (11)
21–30%	20% (11)	2% (1)
31–50%	21% (12)	0%
51–75%	16% (9)	0%

Note: Self-pay includes charity and uninsured.
$p < 0.01$, $X^2 = 52$, DF = 5.

majority of responding hospitals provide public services such as homeless outreach, child care, and counseling for domestic violence. The majority of these hospitals also own major components of integrated health delivery systems, such as community health centers and public health clinics. These hospitals increasingly use case management for managing health care delivery. In general, most urban-based hospitals have salaried physicians. These hospitals do not generally report drastic changes in the past two years. It is of significance, however, that most of these hospitals report a decrease in available funds for financing uninsured patients. At the same time, most of them have experienced no change in the volume of high-risk patients. These hospitals do forecast improvements in infrastructure, primary care capacity, and community facility developments, but foresee reductions in residency programs, non-physician staff, and beds.

Findings corroborate the thesis that these urban-based hospitals, particularly public or safety net hospitals, have been pivotal in the care for residents of the inner cities. Due to their location, ownership of delivery services, assistance services, and adaptation to community needs and service for difficult-to-treat patients, these hospitals play key roles in providing health access to the poor and the underserved in the inner cities. Clearly it is important for managed care organizations to avail themselves of these rich experiences and competency, through collaborations or substantive relationships with these hospitals, as they move into the inner cities. In this way, managed care organizations can become part of the community's safety net.

In terms of graduate medical education, the one key factor affecting the need for increasing residency programs is the need for primary care physicians. However, federal or state actions and market changes negatively influence the size of certain residency programs. The majority of hospitals have not experienced changes in the size of key residency programs.

These findings point out that the evolution of managed care in the inner city is gradually having an impact on medical teaching. Although responding hospitals report that market forces, especially managed care, affect these programs, broad changes in the graduate medical education are not evident. As we argue in this book, the challenges these programs face are important because of managed care's core emphasis on specialty care when the need in the community is clearly for primary care training. Moreover, these programs must be reorganized to adjust academic goals to the structural demands of managed care organizations. This argument is supported by the findings: most of the responding hospitals view the market as a potential negative force in expanding residency programs.

Findings show that the majority of responding urban-based hospitals are operating in either consolidated (40 percent, 46 of 115) or loose and unstructured markets (44 percent, 50 of 115). The percentage and number of responding urban-based hospitals operating in managed markets is therefore comparatively small: 14 percent (16 of 115). In the Northeast, 2 private hospitals report being in a managed market. In the North-Central, only 1 private health system operates in a managed market. In the South, there are 2 urban-based hospitals (private and public) operating in a managed market.

However, in the West, 11 urban-based hospitals (8 public and 3 private) operate in a managed market. Hospitals in managed markets are predominantly in the western region.

These results suggest that managed care is new to the inner city. The rate of evolution of managed care in the inner city is directly related to the ecology of the inner city. The inner-city environment is challenging because of the concentration of poverty and social disadvantage. The needs of the inner-city communities are much broader than the narrow scope of managed care services. As managed care organizations evolve in the inner cities, they will need to address the extent to which they would assume responsibility for addressing some of these social as well as medical needs.

These findings also allow us to examine structural effects of managed care. Most urban-based hospitals do not own a managed care plan and cited the high cost of services as impeding expansion of managed care. This is significant because these hospitals are generally shifting from large acute care services, the focal point for the delivery of care, to delivery systems that are increasingly reliant on the provision of more primary and preventive care in outpatient settings. The high cost of services would slow this realignment by hospitals; this is one of the challenges facing the traditional providers of care. A majority of urban-based hospitals have not experienced any structural effects of managed care in several areas of hospital utilization as yet and do not derive the bulk of their revenues from managed care. These findings strengthen the fact that the evolution of managed care in the inner city is gradual.

Results of the selective bivariate analyses point out significant differences between urban-based public and private hospitals. These findings generally suggest that urban-based public hospitals are lagging behind their private counterparts when it comes to adjusting to managed care. Findings show that there are more private hospitals owning physician practices in the community and contracting with managed care on a noncapitated basis. This means that there are more private hospitals providing physician accessibility as well as minimizing risk in managed care contracts than public hospitals.

Moreover, in 1996, proportionately more private hospitals derived considerable portions of their revenues from managed care, while a greater proportion of public hospitals derived patient charges from self-pay, charity, or uninsured patients. It is clear from these findings that public and private hospitals are adapting to managed care in the inner city differently. In general, due to their safety net functions (provision of care to difficult-to-treat populations and higher margins of indigent and charity care), public hospitals may find it more difficult to adjust to the austere principles of fiscal responsibility dictated by managed care. It is palpable from these findings, however, that public hospitals are aware of the need to adjust organizational structures soon to the demands of the managed market.

References

Agency for Toxic Substances and Disease Registry. *The Nature and Extent of Lead Poisoning in Children in the United States: A Report to Congress.* Washington, D.C.: Agency for Toxic Substances and Disease Registry, 1988.

American Medical Association. "Troublesome Transition: Los Angeles Struggles Despite HMO Experience." *American Medical News,* 1997, 40, 1, 11.

Andrulis, D. *The Urban Health Penalty: New Dimensions and Directions in Inner-City Health Care.* Public Policy Paper 1. Philadelphia: American College of Physicians, 1997.

Andrulis, D., Acuff, K., Weiss, K., and Anderson, R. "Public Hospitals and Health Reform: Choices and Challenges." *American Journal of Public Health,* 1996, 86, 162–165.

Andrulis, D., and Goodman, N. *The Social and Health Landscape of Urban America.* Chicago: American Hospital Publishing, 1999.

Andrulis, D., Shaw-Taylor, Y., Ginsberg, C., and Martin, V. *Urban Social Health: A Chartbook Profiling the Nation's One Hundred Largest Cities.* Washington, D.C.: National Public Health and Hospital Institute, 1995.

Ards, S., and Mincy, R. "Neighborhood Ecology." In D. Besharov (ed.), *When Drug Addicts Have Children.* Washington, D.C.: Child Welfare League of America, 1994.

Association of American Medical Colleges. *National Resident Matching Program.* Washington, D.C.: Association of American Medical Colleges, 1996.

Bashshur, R., Homan, R., and Smith, D. "Beyond the Uninsured: Problems in Access to Care." *Medical Care,* 1994, 32, 409–419.

Bennett, W. J., and Young, G. J. "Fast, Flexible, and Fluid: The Continuing Success of the Charlotte-Mecklenburg Hospital Authority in an Era of Public Hospital Crisis." *Journal of Health Care Finance,* 1997, 23, 51–59.

Bindman, A., and others. "Selection and Exclusion of Primary Care Physicians by Managed Care Organizations." *Journal of the American Medical Association,* 1998, 279, 675–679.

Bischoff, R. O., and others. "Bridging the Gap Between Managed Care and Academic Medicine: An Innovative Fellowship." *American Journal of Managed Care,* 1997, 3, 107–111.

Blendon, R., Aiken, L., Freeman, H., and Corey, C. "Access to Medical Care for Black and White Americans." *Journal of the American Medical Association*, 1989, *261*, 278–281.

Bodenheimer, T. "The HMO Backlash—Righteous or Reactionary?" *New England Journal of Medicine*, 1995, *333*, 1601–1603.

Bograd, H., and others. "Extending Health Maintenance Organization Insurance to the Uninsured." *Journal of the American Medical Association*, 1997, *277*, 1067–1072.

Buerhaus, P. I., and Staiger, D. O. "Managed Care and the Nurse Workforce." *Journal of the American Medical Association*, 1996, *276*, 1487–1493.

Burns, J. B. *Anti-Violent Crime Initiative Fact Sheet*. Chicago: American Medical Association, Northern District of Illinois, 1996.

Burrow, G. "Tensions Within the Academic Health Center." *Academic Medicine*, 1993, *68*, 585–587.

Burstin, H. R., Lipsitz, S. R., and Brennan, T. A. "Socioeconomic Status and Risk for Substantial Medical Care." *Journal of the American Medical Association*, 1992, *268*, 2382–2387.

Butterfield, F. "Crime Keeps on Falling, But Prisons Keep on Filling." *New York Times Week in Review*, Sept. 28, 1997, p. 1.

Caper, S., and Fargason, C. "A Way to Approach the Strategic Decisions Facing Academic Health Centers." *Academic Medicine*, 1996, *71*, 337–342.

Center for Workforce Studies, University at Albany. *The Changing Health Care System in New York City: Implications for the Health Workforce*. Albany, N.Y.: Century Concepts, May 1997.

Centers for Disease Control and Prevention. "Poverty and Infant Mortality—United States, 1988." *Morbidity and Mortality Weekly Report*, 1995, *44*, 922–927.

Centerwall, B. "Race, Socioeconomic Status and Domestic Homicide." *Journal of the American Medical Association*, 1995, *273*, 1755–1758.

Clayton, L., and Byrd, M. "The African-American Cancer Crisis, Part I: The Problem." *Journal of Health Care for the Poor and Underserved*, 1993, *4*, 83–101.

"Clinics Losing Ground in Drive Toward Managed Care." *Washington Post*, Jan. 3, 1998.

Coughlin, T., Rajan, S., Zuckerman, S., and Marsteller, J. *Health Policy for Low-Income People in Minnesota*. Washington, D.C.: Urban Institute, 1997.

Council on Ethical and Judicial Affairs. "Black-White Disparities in Health Care." *Journal of the American Medical Association*, May 2, 1990, pp. 2344–2346.

Douglass, R., and Torres, R. "Evaluation of a Managed Care Program for the Non-Medicaid Urban Poor." *Journal of Health Care for the Poor and Underserved*, 1994, *5*, 83–97.

Ellwood, M., and Ku, L. "Welfare and Immigration Reforms: Unintended Side Effects for Medicaid." *Health Affairs*, 1998, *17*, 137–151.

Fein, O. "The Influence of Social Class on Health Status: American and British Research on Health Inequalities." *Journal of General Internal Medicine*, 1995, *10*, 577–586.

Feldman, J. G., Minkoff, H. L., McCalla, S., and Salwen, M. "A Cohort Study of the Impact of Perinatal Drug Use on Prematurity in an Inner-City Population." *American Journal of Public Health*, 1992, *82*, 726–728.

Foltin, G. "Critical Issues in Urban Emergency Medical Services for Children." *Pediatrics*, 1995 (Suppl.), *96*, 174–179.

"For Millions of Americans, English Is a Second Language." *New York Times*, Apr. 28, 1997, p. 1.

Foreman, S. "Social Responsibility and the Academic Medical Center: Building Community-Based Systems for the Nation's Health." *Academic Medicine*, 1994, *69*, 97–102.

Fossett, J., and Perloff, J. *The "New" Health Reform and Access to Care: The Problem of the Inner City*. Washington, D.C.: Kaiser Commission of the Future of Medicaid, 1995.

Fox, P., and Fama, T. "Managed Care and Chronic Illness: An Overview." *Managed Care Quarterly*, 1996, *4*, 1–4.

Franks, P., Clancy, G., and Gold, M. "Health Insurance and Mortality." *Journal of the American Medical Association*, 1993, *270*, 737–741.

Freeman, H. "The Health of Adults." Paper presented at Health Care in Underserved Urban America: Implications for Health Reform, Columbia University, June 7–8, 1993.

Freundberg, N. *Health Promotion in the City*. New York: Hunter College, 1997.

Fried, B. M., and Besdine, R. W. "A Perspective on Academic Medicine from the Nation's Largest Managed Care Purchaser." *Academic Medicine*, 1996, *7*, 260–261.

Friedman, E. "California Public Hospitals: The Buck Has Stopped." *Journal of the American Medical Association*, 1997a, *277*, 577–581.

Friedman, E. "Managed Care and Medical Education: Hard Cases and Hard Choices." *Academic Medicine*, 1997b, *72*, 325–331.

Friedman, N. "Diabetes and Managed Care: The Lovelace Health System's Episode of Care Treatment." *Managed Care Quarterly*, 1996, *4*, 43–49.

Fubani, S. "Where's the 'Uninsurance Epidemic'?" *Healthcare Trends Report*, 1997, *11*, 1–2.

Gage, L., and others. *America's Essential Providers*. Washington, D.C.: National Association of Public Hospitals, 1996.

Gales, S. E. "Managed Community Health: An Integrated Model Journal of Health Care." *Finance*, 1996, *23*, 48–56.

Garfield, R., Broe, D., and Albano, B. "The Role of Academic Medical Centers in Delivery of Primary Care: An Urban Study." *Academic Medicine*, 1995, *70*, 405–409.

Gaskins, D. J., Hadley, J., and Freeman, V. G. *Are Urban Safety Net Hospitals Losing the Competition for Low-Risk Medicaid Patients?* Washington, D.C.:

Institute for Health Care Research and Policy, Georgetown University Medical Center, June 1998.

Gautam, K., Arrington, F., and Campbell, C. "Inner-City Hospitals: A Call for Research." *Journal of Health Care for the Poor and Underserved*, 1995, 6, 387–403.

Gelberg, L., Doblin, B., and Leake, B. "Ambulatory Health Services Provided to Low-Income and Homeless Adult Patients in a Major Community Health Center." *Journal of General Internal Medicine*, 1996, 11, 156–162.

GHAA and KPMG. *Serving Vulnerable Populations: HMOs and Essential Community Providers*. Washington, D.C.: GHAA and KPMG Peat Marwick, Aug. 12, 1994.

Ginsberg, C., Benesch, B., and Bennett, B. *Violence in the United States—Characteristics and Issues for Safety Net Health System*. Washington, D.C.: National Association of Public Hospitals and Health Systems, 1997.

Gold, M. *Contemporary Managed Care*. Chicago: Health Administration Press, 1998.

Gold, M., Frazer, H., and Schoen, C. *Managed Care and Low Income Populations: A Case Study of Managed Care in Tennessee*. Washington, D.C.: Kaiser Family Foundation and the Commonwealth Fund, July 1995.

Goldman, B. "Improving Access to the Underserved Through Medicaid Managed Care. *Journal of Health Care for the Poor and Underserved*, 1993, 4, 290–298.

Goldstein, A. "Clinics Losing Ground in Drive Toward Managed Care." *Washington Post*, Jan. 3, 1998, p. A–01.

"Government Lags in Steps to Widen Health Coverage." *New York Times*, Aug. 9, 1998, p. 1.

Greenberg, M. "American Cities: Good and Bad News About Public Health." *Bulletin of the New York Academy of Medicine*, 1991, 67, 17–21.

Greineder, D. K. "The Adaptation of Asthma Practice Guidelines into Clinical Care: The Harvard Pilgrim Health Care Experience." *Journal of Outcomes Management*, 1996, pp. 4–9.

Grisso, J., Schwarz, D., Miles, C., and Holmes, J. "Injuries Among Inner-City Minority Women: A Population-Based Longitudinal Study." *American Journal of Public Health*, 1996, 86, 67–70.

Grumbach, K., Vranizan, K., and Bindman, A. B. "Physician Supply and Access to Care in Urban Communities." *Health Affairs*, 1997, 16, 71–86.

Hadley, J., Steinburg, E. P., and Feder, J. "Comparison of Uninsured and Privately Insured Hospital Patients: Condition on Admission, Resources Use, and Outcome." *Journal of the American Medical Association*, 1991, 265, 374–379.

Halverson, P., and others. "Managed Care: The Public Health Challenge of TB." *Public Health Reports*, 1997, 112, 22–28.

Hamburg, B. "Issues in Urban Health, in Health Care in Underserved Urban America: Implications for National Health Reform." Paper presented at Health Care in Underserved Urban America: Implications for Health Reform, Columbia University, June 7–8, 1993.

Harris, J., and Havemann, J. "Welfare Rolls Continue Sharp Decline." *Washington Post*, Aug. 13, 1997, p.1.

Harris, J. R., and others. "Prevention and Managed Care: Opportunities for Managed Care Organizations, Purchasers of Health Care, and Public Health Agencies." *HMO Practice*, 1996, *10*, 24–27.

Hart, G., and others. "Physician Staffing Ratios in Staff Model HMOs." *Health Affairs*, 1997, *16*, 55–69.

Hayward, R. A., Shapiro, M. F., Freeman, H. E., and Corey, C. "Inequities in Health Services Among Insured Americans: Do Working-Age Adults Have Less Access to Medical Care Than the Elderly?" *New England Journal of Medicine*, 1988, *318*, 1507–1512.

"Health Gap Grows, with Black Americans Trailing Whites, Studies Say." *New York Times*, Jan. 26, 1998, p. A16.

"Health Insurers Seek Big Increases in Their Premiums." *New York Times*, Apr. 24, 1998, p. 1.

Henley, A. J., and Clifford, M. C. "Managed Health Care for Medicaid Enrollees: The Philadelphia Model." *Journal of Health Care for the Poor and Underserved*, 1993, *4*, 210–217.

Hillman, A. L., Goldfarb, N., Eisenberg, J. M., and Kelley, M. A. "An Academic Medical Center's Experience with Mandatory Managed Care for Medicaid Recipients." *Academic Medicine*, 1991, *66*, 134–138.

"HIP to Offer Free Childhood Immunizations." *HMO Managers Letter*, Apr. 19, 1993.

Hospitals and Health Networks. Jan. 5, 1996.

Hospitals Magazine. May 5, 1993.

"Hospitals Serving the Poor Struggle to Retain Patients." *New York Times*, Sept. 3, 1997, p. 1.

Hurley, R., and McCue, M. *Medicaid and Commercial HHMs: An At-Risk Relationship*. Princeton, N.J.: Robert Wood Johnson Foundation, Medicaid Managed Care Program, May 1998.

Hurley, R., and Walin, S. *Adopting and Adapting Managed Care for Medicaid Beneficiaries: An Imperfect Transition*. Occasional paper no. 7. Washington, D.C.: Urban Institute, 1998.

Hurley, R., Zinn, J., Rosko, M., and Kuder, J. *Adapting to Mandatory Medicaid Managed Care: Preparations and Perspectives Among Community Health Providers*. Philadelphia: Pew Charitable Trusts, 1997.

Hutson, H., and others. "The Epidemic of Gang-Related Homicides in Los Angeles County from 1979 Through 1994." *Journal of the American Medical Association*, 1995, *274*, 1031–1036.

"In Medicine, Government Rises Again." *New York Times Week in Review*, Dec. 7, 1997, p. 1.

Jacobs, S. "Using Research for Successful Medicare and Medicaid Risk Marketing." *Managed Care Quarterly*, 1996, 4(4), 30.

Jaklevic, M. "Managed Indigent Care." *Modern Health Care*, 1997, 27, 44.

Kahn, K., and others. "Health Care for Black and Poor Hospitalized Medicare Patients." *Journal of the American Medical Association*, 1994, 271, 1169–1174.

Keane, V., and others. "Perceptions of Vaccine Efficacy, Illness, and Health Among Inner-City Parents." *Clinical Pediatrics*, 1993, 32, 2–7.

Kindig, D., and others. "Trends in Medical Availability in 10 Urban Areas from 1963–1980." *Inquiry*, 1987, 24, 136–1146.

Kizer, K., Vasser, M., Harry, R., and Layton, K. "Hospitalization Charges, Costs and Income for Firearm-Related Injuries at a University Trauma Center." *Journal of the American Medical Association*, 1995, 273, 1768–1773.

Klein, M., and Maxson, C. "Street Gang Violence." In N. A. Weiner and M. E. Wolfgang (eds.), *Violent Crime, Violent Criminals*. Thousand Oaks, Calif.: Sage, 1989.

Kogan, M. D., Kotelchuck, M., Alexander, G. R., and Johnson, W. E. "Racial Disparities in Reported Prenatal Care Advice from Health Care Providers." *American Journal of Public Health*, 1994, 84, 82–88.

Komaromy, M., and others. "The Role of Black and Hispanic Physicians in Providing Care for Underserved Populations." *New England Journal of Medicine*, 1996, 334, 1305–1310.

Koop, C. E., and Lundberg, G. D. "Violence in America: A Public Health Emergency." *Journal of the American Medical Association*, 1992, 267, 3075–3076.

Koplan, J. (ed.). "Special Challenge of Prevention in the Inner-City." Paper presented at Health Care in Underserved Urban America: Implications for Health Reform, Columbia University, June 7–8, 1993.

Lang, D., and Polansky, M. "Pattern of Asthma Mortality in Philadelphia from 1969–1991." *New England Journal of Medicine*, 1994, 331, 1542–1546.

Lantz, P., and others. "Socioeconomic Factors, Health Behaviors, and Mortality." *Journal of the American Medical Association*, 1998, 279, 1703–1708.

"Largest HMOs Cutting the Poor and the Elderly." *New York Times*, July 1998.

Lawrence, L. "Health-Care Reform and the Urban Condition." *Journal of the National Medical Association*, 1994, 86, 100–102.

Levine, D. M., and others. "Community-Academic Health Center Partnerships for Underserved Minority Populations: One Solution to a National Crisis." *Journal of the American Medical Association*, 1994, 272, 309–311.

Lillie-Blanton, M., and Lyons, B. "Managed Care and Low-Income Populations: Recent State Experiences." *Health Affairs*, 1998, 17, 238–247.

Link, B., and others. "Lifetime and Five-Year Prevalence of Homelessness in the United States." *American Journal of Public Health*, 1994, 4, 1907–1912.

Loughlin, J., Bronner, E., and Mascare, J. "Women's Health Services: Restructuring for Medicaid Managed Care." *Journal of Ambulatory Care Management,* 1997, *21,* 70–77.

"Low Medicaid Fees Seen Depriving the Poor of Care." *New York Times,* Apr. 2, 1991, p. 1.

Managed Care Monitor. "Teaching Hospitals: Managed Care Creates Obstacles, American Healthline." *National Journal,* May 20, 1997.

McCord, C., and Freeman, H. "Excess Mortality in Harlem." *New England Journal of Medicine,* 1990, *322,* 173–179.

McFadden, E. R., and Gilbert, I. A. "Asthma." *New England Journal of Medicine,* 1992, *327,* 1928–1935.

McGuire, D. "Huge Jumps in Medicaid Managed Care Means Opportunity for MCOs." *Managed Care Outlook,* 1996, *9,* 1–2.

McManus, M. A., and Fox, H. B. "Enhancing Preventive and Primary Care for Children with Chronic or Disabling Conditions Served in Health Maintenance Organizations." *Managed Care Quarterly,* 1996, *4,* 19–29.

Marquis, S., and Long, S. "Reconsidering the Effect of Medicaid on Health Care Service Use." *Health Services Research,* 1996, *30,* 791–808.

Master, R. J. "Pneumocystis Pneumonia in a Prepaid Care System Caring for a Medicaid-Covered Population with AIDs." *Journal of Ambulatory Care Management,* 1996, *19,* 38–45.

Medicaid Access Study Group. "Access of Medicaid Recipients to Outpatient Care." *New England Journal of Medicine,* 1994, *330,* 1426–1430.

Mendoza, F. "The Health of Latino Children in the United States." *Current Problems in Pediatrics,* 1995, *25,* 310.

Musto, D. *The American Disease: Origins of Narcotic Control.* Oxford: Oxford University Press, 1987.

National Association of Community Health Centers. *Progress Report 1995.* Washington, D.C.: National Association of Community Health Centers, 1995.

National Association of Public Hospitals and Health Systems. *Findings from the 1996 NAPH Hospital Characteristics Survey.* Washington, D.C.: National Association of Public Hospitals and Health Systems, Apr. 1998.

National Center for Children in Poverty. *News and Issues,* Winter–Spring 1995, *5*(1).

National Center for Health Statistics. *Health, United States.* Washington, D.C.: National Center for Health Statistics, 1994.

National Center for Health Statistics. *Ambulatory Care Visits for Asthma: United States 1993–94.* Advanced Data Report No. 277. Washington, D.C.: U.S. National Center for Health Statistics, 1996.

Nelson, K., Brown, M., and Lurie, N. "Hunger in an Adult Patient Population." *Journal of the American Medical Association,* 1998, *279,* 1211–1214.

Nichols, L., Ku, L. Norton, S., and Wall, S. *Health Policy for Low-Income People in Washington.* Washington, D.C.: Urban Institute, 1997.

Nordin, J., Rolnick, S., and Griffin, J. "Prevalence of Excess Lead Absorption and Associated Risk Factors in Children Enrolled in a Midwestern Health Maintenance Organization." *Pediatrics,* 1994, *93,* 172–177.

Oakie, S. "Study Links Cancer, Poverty: Blacks' Higher Rates Are Tied to Income." *Washington Post,* Apr. 17, 1991.

Oden, C. W. "Managed Care and Health Care Services to Urban/Inner City Communities: The Watts Health Foundation, Inc. Experience." Testimony Before the Finance Committee, U.S. Senate. Apr. 21, 1994.

Orbovich, C. "Collaborative Strategies for Success in the Changing Medicaid Market: The Perspectives of Community-Based Providers and Managed Care Organizations." Prepared for the American Association of Health Plans and the Health Resources and Services Administration Conference: Collaborative Strategies for Success in the Changing Medicaid Market, Washington, D.C., Apr. 1–2, 1996.

Page, L. "Moving Away from Medicaid." *AMA News,* June 1, 1998.

Pardes, H. "The Future of Medical Schools and Teaching Hospitals in the Era of Managed Care." *Academic Medicine,* 1997, *72,* 97–102.

Parker, S., Greer, S., and Zuckerman, B. "Double Jeopardy: The Impact of Poverty on Early Child Development." *Pediatric Clinics of North America,* 1988, *35,* 1227–1240.

Peat Marwick. *Serving Vulnerable Populations: HMOs and Essential Community Providers.* Washington, D.C.: Peat Marwick, 1994.

Peck, M., and Hubbert, E. (eds.). *Changing the Rules: Medicaid Managed Care and MCH in U.S. Cities.* Special Report I. Omaha: CityMatch, 1994.

Perloff, J., Kletke, P., Fossett, J., and Banks, S. "Medicaid Participation Among Urban Primary Care Physicians." *Medical Care,* 1997, *35,* 142–147.

Physician Payment Review Commission. *Models of Care for Inner City Populations.* Selected External Research Series No. 2. Washington, D.C.: Physician Payment Review Commission, Dec. 1994.

Pinner, R., and others. "Trends in Infectious Diseases, Mortality in the United States." *Journal of the American Medical Association,* 1996, *27,* 189–193.

Polednak, A. "Poverty, Residential Segregation and Black/White Mortality in Urban Areas." *Journal of Health Care for the Poor and Underserved,* 1993, *4,* 363–373.

Politzer, B. "Member Appeal." *HMO Magazine,* 1995, *36,* 23–29.

Politzer, R., Harris, D., Gaston, M., and Mullen, P. "Primary Care Physician Supply and the Medically Underserved." *Journal of the American Medical Association,* 1991, *26,* 104–109.

Pope, T. "United Health Plan Bridges Gap Between HMOs and Community Health Centers." *HMO Practice,* 1995, *9,* 71–74.

Quint, J., Bos, J., and Polit, D. *New Chance: Final Report on a Comprehensive Program for Young Mothers in Poverty and Their Children*. New York: Manpower Demonstration Research Corporation, Oct. 1997.

Rask, K., Williams, M., Parker, R., and McNagny, S. "Obstacles Predicting Lack of a Regular Provider and Delays in Seeking Care for Patients at an Urban Public Hospital." *Journal of the American Medical Association*, 1994, *271*, 1931–1933.

Reddington, T., Lippincott, J., Lindsay, D., and Wones, R. "How an Academic Health Center and a Community Health Center Found Common Ground" *Academic Medicine*, 1995, *70*, 21–26.

Reiss, A. J., and Roth, J. A. (eds.). *Understanding and Preventing Violence*. Washington, D.C.: National Academy Press, 1993.

Renneker, M., and others. "An Inner-City Cancer Prevention Clinic in West Oakland." *Cancer Practice*, 1994, *2*, 427–437.

Reuter, J. *The Financing of Academic Health Centers: A Chart Book*. (Research supported by the Commonwealth Fund.) Washington, D.C.: Institute for Health Care Research and Policy, Georgetown University, 1997a.

Reuter, J. *Understanding the Social Missions of Academic Health Centers*. New York: Commonwealth Fund Task Force, 1997b.

Rivo, M., and Satcher, D. "Improving Access to Health Care Through Physician Workforce Reform." *Journal of the American Medical Association*, 1993, *270*(9), 1074–1078.

Robinson, J. "Decline in Hospital Utilization and Cost Inflation Under Managed Care in California." *Journal of the American Medical Association*, 1996, *276*, 1060–1064.

Ropp, L., Visintainer, P., Uman, J., and Treloar, D. "Death in the City: An American Childhood Tragedy." *Journal of the American Medical Association*, 1995, *267*, 3075–3076.

Rosenstreich, D. L., and others. "The Role of Cockroach Allergy and Exposure to Cockroach Allergen in Causing Morbidity Among Inner-City Children with Asthma." *New England Journal of Medicine*, 1997, *336*, 1356–1363.

Rowland, D., Rosenbaum, S., Simon, L., and Chait, E. *Medicaid and Managed Care: Lessons from the Literature*. Washington, D.C.: Kaiser Commission on the Future of Medicaid, Mar. 1995.

Sabol, B. "The Urban Child." *Journal of Health Care for the Poor and Underserved*, 1991, *2*(1), 59–73.

Salit, S., and others. "Hospitalization Costs Associated with Homelessness in New York City." *New England Journal of Medicine*, 1998, *338*, 1734–1740.

Sandman, D., Schoen, C., DesRoches, C., and Makonnen, M. *The Commonwealth Fund Survey of Health Care in New York City*. New York: Commonwealth Fund, 1998.

Sayer, B., and Peterfreund, N. "Insurance, Income, and Access to Ambulatory Care in King County, Washington." *American Journal of Public Health,* 1993, *83,* 1583–1587.

Schauffler, H., and Wolin, J. "Community Health Clinics Under Managed Competition: Navigating Unchartered Waters." *Health Politics, Policy and Law,* 1996, *21,* 461–488.

Scott-Collins, K., Schoen, C., and Sandman, D. R. *The Commonwealth Fund Survey of Physician Experiences with Managed Care.* New York: Commonwealth Fund, Mar. 1997.

Selik, R., Chu, S., and Buehler, J. "HIV Infection as Leading Cause of Death Among Young Adults in U.S. Cities and States." *Journal of the American Medical Association,* 1993, *269,* 2991–2994.

Shi, L. "The Relationship Between Primary Care and Life Chances." *Journal of Health Care for the Poor and Underserved,* 1992, *3,* 321–325.

Shoemaker, W., and others. "Urban Violence in Los Angeles in the Aftermath of the Riots." *Journal of the American Medical Association,* 1993, *270,* 2833–2837.

Showstack, J., and others. "Health of the Public: The Private Sector Challenge." *Journal of the American Medical Association,* 1996, *276,* 1071–1074.

Singer, M. "AIDS and the Health Crisis of the U.S. Urban Poor: The Perspective of Critical Medical Anthropology." *Social Science and Medicine,* 1994, *39,* 931–948.

Singh, G., and Yu, S. "US Childhood Mortality, 1950 Through 1993: Trends and Socioeconomic Differentials." *American Journal of Public Health,* 1996, *86,* 505–512.

Smith, G., and others. "Socioeconomic Differentials in Mortality Risk Among Men Screened for Multiple Risk Factor Intervention Trial I: White Men." *American Journal of Public Health,* 1996, *86,* 497–504.

Spergel, I. "Survey." National Youth Gang Supression and Intervention Program. Chicago: School of Social Service, University of Chicago, 1989.

Spergel, I. *The Youth Gang Problem: A Community Approach.* New York: Oxford University Press. 1995.

Spillman, B. "The Impact of Being Uninsured on Utilization of Basic Health Care Services." *Inquiry,* 1992, *29,* 457–466.

State Health Watch. "Interview with Colleen Kivlahan: Missouri Carves Out Public Health to Safeguard Medicaid Population During Shift to Managed Care." Dec. 1995, pp. 5–6.

State Health Watch. "Texas Hospital Offers Managed Care to Uninsured." Jun. 1997, p. 5.

Steinberg, C., and Baxter, R. "Accountable Communities: How Norms and Values Affect Health System Change." *Health Affairs,* 1998, *17,* 149–157.

Studnicki, J., and others. "Analyzing Organizational Practices in Local Health Departments." *Public Health Report,* 1994, *109,* 485–490.

Theide, K., and others. "Who Is Still Uninsured in Minnesota?" *Journal of the American Medical Association* 1997, *278*, 1191–1195.

Their, S. "Academic Medicine's Choice in an Era of Reform." *Academic Medicine*, 1994, *69*, 185–189.

U.S. Department of Health and Human Services, Bureau of Primary Care. *Selected Statistics on Health Professional Shortage Areas.* Washington, D.C.: U.S. Government Printing Office, 1993a.

U.S. Department of Health and Human Services, Office of Inspector General. *School-Based Health Centers and Managed Care.* OEI–05–92–00680. Washington, D.C.: U.S. Government Printing Office, 1993b.

U.S. General Accounting Office. *Healthpass: An Evaluation of a Managed Care Program for Certain Philadelphia Residents.* Washington, D.C.: U.S. Government Printing Office, May 1993.

U.S. General Accounting office. *Community Health Centers: Challenges in Transition to Prepaid Managed Care.* Washington, D.C.: Government Printing Office, May 1995.

Veloski, J., and others. "Medical Student Education in Managed Care Settings: Beyond HMOs." *Journal of the American Medical Association*, 1996, *276*, 667–671.

Wallace, D. "Roots of Increased Health Care Inequality in New York." *Social Science and Medicine*, 1990, *31*, 1219–1227.

Wallace, R., Huang, Y., Gould, P., and Wallace, D. "The Hierarchical Diffusion of AIDS and Violent Crime Among U.S. Metropolitan Regions: Inner City Decay, Stochastic Resonance and Reversal of the Mortality Transition." *Social Science and Medicine*, forthcoming.

Ware, J., and others. "Differences in Four-Year Health Outcomes for Elderly and Indigent, Chronically Ill Patients Treated in HMO and Fee-for-Service Systems." *Journal of the American Medical Association*, 1996, *276*, 1039–1047.

Weissman, J. "Uncompensated Hospital Care: Will It Be There If We Need It?" *Journal of the American Medical Association*, 1996, *276*, 823–828.

Weissman, J., and Epstein, A. M. "Case Mix and Resource Utilization by Uninsured Hospitalized Patients in the Boston Metropolitan Area." *Journal of the American Medical Association*, 1989, *261*, 3572–3576.

Welch, W. P., and Wade, M. "The Relative Cost of Medicaid Enrollees and the Commercially Insured in HMOs." *Health Affairs*, 1995, *14*, 212–223.

Williams, L. *Mourning in America: Health Problems, Mortality, and Homelessness.* Washington, D.C.: National Coalition for the Homeless, 1991.

Wilson, W. *The Truly Disadvantaged.* Chicago: University of Chicago Press, 1987.

Wise, P. "Infant Mortality as a Social Mirror." *New England Journal of Medicine*, 1992, *326*, 1558–1560.

Witek, J. E., and Hostage, J. L. "Medicaid Managed Care: Problems and Promise." *Journal of Ambulatory Care Management*, 1994, *17*, 61–69.

Zall, R. "Observations on Current Threats and Future Prospects Facing the Health Care Safety Net." *Grantmakers in Health Issue Dialogue: Health Philanthropy and the Safety Net,* Chicago, July 31, 1996.

Zollinger, T. W., Saywell, R. M., Jr., and Chu, D. K. "Uncompensated Hospital Care for Pregnancy and Childbirth Cases." *American Journal of Public Health,* 1991, *81,* 1017–1022.

Index

A

Academic health centers (AHCs): case management in, 78; community health center alliances with, 73; community health centers subsumed under, 62–63; educational mission of, 79–81, 84; funding of, 68–69; issues of, in managed care environment, 68–72; managed care fellowships of, 49; managed care integration of, 67–84; management approaches of, 72–73; missions of, 67, 68, 78, 82, 83, 113; organizational redirection of, 74–76, 94–95; research mission of, 79–83, 84; specialty services of, 81–83, 84; uncompensated care burden of, 70–72. *See also* Teaching hospitals

Academic medicine inertia, 81

Access to health care: inner-city environment and, 10–22; insurance and, 15–18; managed care implementation and, 45–49; managed care outcomes for, 26–28; for Medicaid enrollees, 17, 27, 85–86; minority status and, 14–15, 48; physician supply and, 18–22, 45–49, 65; poverty and, 10–15; quality of care and, 14–15; state regulation of, 106–107; welfare reform and, 18

Acuff, K., 81, 83

Administrative costs: of Medicaid managed care plans, 28; of physicians in multiple managed care plans, 47

Adverse selection, 88–90, 98

Affirmative action, 22, 66

African Americans: disease among, 12–13; disproportionate incarceration of male, 9; lack of insurance of, 15; life expectancy of, 12; mortality and violence among young, 8, 9; mortality rates of, 12–13; poverty segregation of, 12; prenatal counseling of, 6; quality of care for, 14; substance abuse among, 13

Agency for Toxic Substances and Disease Registry, 8

AIDS: case management for, 78; homelessness and, 4; inner-city environment and, 5; minority status and, 13; targeted intervention for, 34

Aiken, L., 12, 14

Alaska, 85

Albuquerque, New Mexico, 33–34

Alcohol advertising, 2

Alcoholism: health problems of, 6, 7, 13; homelessness and, 4; minority status and, 13. *See also* Substance abuse

Alexander, G. R., 6

Allied health professionals, 45–49. *See also* Physicians

Ambulatory care arrangements, 76

American Association of Health Plans, 50

American Cancer Society, 35–36

American Hospital Association (AHA), 95

American Medical Association (AMA), 28, 46; Council on Ethical and Judicial Affairs, 9, 12, 15; Physician Master File, 47

AT&T language banks, 32

Anderson, R., 81, 83

Andrulis, D., 6, 7, 8, 81, 83

Angiography, 14

Anterior myocardial infarction, 14

Archibishop's Commission on Community Health, St. Louis, 41

Ards, S., 11, 12

Asian-Pacific Islanders, 13

Printed and bound by CPI Group (UK) Ltd, Croydon, CR0 4YY

16/04/2025

14658442-0001